newest ed.
JmC nov. 2011

Principles of Perioperative Practice

For Churchill Livingstone:

Commissioning Editor: Ninette Premdas
Project Development Manager: Katrina Mather
Project Manager: Jane Shanks
Design Direction: George Ajayi

Principles of Perioperative Practice

Edited by

Martin Hind MSc BSc(Hons) PGDE DPSN RGN RNT
Senior Lecturer in Critical Care, Institute of Health and Community Studies,
Bournemouth University, UK

Paul Wicker BSc(Nursing) RGN RMN CCNS
(Operating Department Nursing)
Education Coordinator, Theatres, Royal Infirmary of Edinburgh,
Lothian University Hospitals NHS Trust, Edinburgh, UK; Editor,
British Journal of Theatre Nursing

Foreword by

Jane Salvage RGN BA MSc HonLLD
Editor in Chief, *Nursing Times*, London, UK

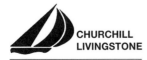CHURCHILL
LIVINGSTONE

EDINBURGH LONDON NEW YORK PHILADELPHIA ST LOUIS SYDNEY TORONTO 2000

CHURCHILL LIVINGSTONE
An imprint of Harcourt Publishers Limited

© Harcourt Publishers Limited 2000

⚡ is a registered trademark of Harcourt Publishers Limited

First published 2000

0 443 06251 X

British Library Cataloguing in Publication Data
A catalogue record for this book is available from the British Library.

Library of Congress Cataloging in Publication Data
A catalog record for this book is available from the Library of Congress.

Note
Medical knowledge is constantly changing. As new information becomes available, changes in treatment, procedures, equipment and the use of drugs become necessary. The editors, contributors and the publishers have, as far as it is possible, taken care to ensure that the information given in this text is accurate and up to date. However, readers are strongly advised to confirm that the information, especially with regard to drug usage, complies with the latest legislation and standards of practice.

The
publisher's
policy is to use
**paper manufactured
from sustainable forests**

Printed in China

Contents

Contributors

Maureen Dyke RGN RM RHV BSc
Anaesthetic Staff Nurse, Theatre Directorate, Royal Cornwall Hospital,
Truro, UK

Martin Hind MSc BSc(Hons) PGDE DPSN RGN RNT
Senior Lecturer in Critical Care, Institute of Health and Community Studies,
Bournemouth University, Dorset, UK

Charles Laugharne BA(Hons) MN MSc RN PGCE RNT
Lecturer in Nursing Studies, University of Wales College of Medicine,
Cardiff, UK

Andy Mardell RGN DipN BN(Hons)
Charge Nurse, Main Theatres, University Hospital of Wales,
Cardiff, UK

Adrienne Montgomery MN(Wales) DipN(Lond) RGON SCM RCNT PhD
candidate(Griffith)
Head of Department, Department of Health Studies, Manukau Institute of
Technology, Auckland, New Zealand

Jane H Reid RGN DPNS BSc(Hons) PGCEA MSc
Senior Lecturer, Perioperative Care, Institute of Health and Community
Studies, Bournemouth University, Dorset, UK

Andrea Star RGN BSc(Hons) CMS
Director of Nursing and Quality, Stirling Royal Infirmary NHS Trust,
Stirling, UK

Marion Taylor RGN DipN BEd(Hons)
Practice Development Nurse, Operating Department, Royal Free Hospital,
London, UK

Sheila Turner MSc(Health) BSc(Hons) RGN
Lecturer Practitioner, Perioperative Nursing,
Florence Nightingale School of Nursing and Midwifery,
King's College University of London and King's
College Hospital, UK

Bernice J M West MA(Hons) RGN PhD PGCert
Director, Centre for Nurse Practice, Research and Development, Robert
Gordon University, Aberdeen, UK

Paul Wicker BSc(Nursing) RGN RMN CCNS(Operating Department
Nursing)

Education Coordinator, Theatres, Royal Infirmary of Edinburgh,
University Hospitals NHS Trust, Edinburgh,
UK; Editor, *British Journal of Perioperative Nursing*

Marilyn Williams RGN DipN BSc(Hons) PGDE
Senior Lecturer, University of Wolverhampton, School of Nursing and
Midwifery, Wolverhampton, UK

Jo Wilson MSc(Dist) PGDip BSc(Hons) MIPD AIRM MHSM RGN RM RSCN
Director of Clinical Services, HRRI, Newcastle upon Tyne, UK

Kate Woodhead RGN DMS
Freelance Operating Theatre Consultant; Chairman of National Association of
Theatre Nurses

Jacqueline F M Younger RGN BSc(Hons)
Education and Development Directorate Manager, Papworth Hospital,
Cambridge, UK

Foreword

Operating departments are the setting for one of the great media clichés. Eyes meet meaningfully over the masks, sweat drips from the surgeon's brow and the super-efficient sister smartly hands him the instruments as he barks his commands. From Mills and Boon to TV soaps, the image is all too familiar.

Like all stereotypes it contains a grain of truth – or at least, it may have once upon a time. This book, however, shows how far nurses have travelled since those distant hierarchical days. Their current concerns range from measuring quality to ethical considerations, and even the 'theatre nurse' title is giving way to the more accurate if less memorable 'perioperative' label. The variety of issues explored in these pages shows the complexity and breadth of the knowledge, skills and values today's perioperative nurse must master to become the consummate professional.

Sadly, the development and nature of this speciality seems to be one of nursing's best kept secrets, and many unenlightened colleagues are still fooled by the stereotype. This may contribute to the recruitment problems highlighted here by Adrienne Montgomery. Only direct experience of the theatre environment can prove its allure, but changes in nursing education mean that most nursing students have little or no exposure to theatres – which is dstroying the tradition of attracting promising novices by inviting them to return once qualified.

I myself managed to avoid the operating department throughout my clinical nursing career. As a student, by the time the option of a placement there arose, I was desperate to escape the hospital, and happily chose a spell in the community instead. Theatres remained a scary environment of which my only experience was as a reluctant patient. Like thousands of other students, no opportunity came along to change my ignorant views.

If I had read this book at that time, I might have had second thoughts. It is a wonderful advertisement for perioperative nursing, as well as a barometer of how nursing is developing and maturing. The issues with which it grapples are central to the profession's future. Take teamwork, roles and relationships. A growing number of operating department practitioners and support workers are being employed to fill the gaps caused by nursing shortages, and in the belief that they are cheaper – though studies tend to show that employing qualified nurses is the cost-effective option. Those staff are also increasingly well educated and beginning to pursue professional status, just as nursing itself did in recent decads. This might be seen as a threat to the traditional nursing role, removing some of its most satisfying aspects, or it can be seen as a way of making best use of scarce nursing skills. Both points of view can be justified, and perhaps both are true.

At the other end of the spectrum, too, one group's opportunity can be seen as a threat to another. In a similar shifting of boundaries, similarly driven by a mixture of logic, idealism and pragmatism, nurses are increasingly undertaking aspects of the traditional medical role. In my experience as a seasoned observer of the health care scene, nowhere have role boundaries been as hotly contested as in anaesthetics. When *Nursing Times* published articles debating the anaesthetic nurse's expanding role, I received some extraordinarily vitriolic correspondence and realised we had stepped into a minefield. Theatres, it seemed, could be more like Roman amphitheatres.

Although the theatre environment stereotypically attracts the most arrogant medical types, it is actually an area where teamwork is essential to success. In many specialities the doctor or nurse practitioner can work effectively alone, but not here. I recently came across a beautiful descritpion of this, not in a textbook but in a diary written by the great British sculptor Barbara Hepworth. Her interest in hospitals was aroused when her child needed surgery, and she watched the operations. She was scared at first, but became enthralled by 'the beauty in the co-ordinated human endeavour in the operating theatre' (Hepworth 1993).

She captured this in exquisite drawings (some now owned by the Royal College of Surgeons) of doctors and nurses in theate, which inspired her later work. 'I became completely absorbed by two things,' Dame Barbara wrote. 'First, the extraordinary beauty of purpose between human beings all dedicated to the saving of life; and second by the way this special grace (of ming and body) indued a . . . kind of abstract sculpture, very close to what I had been seeking in my own work.'

'I wasn't trying to tell a story,' she wrote, 'but no matter how many people were involved, their action and poise and intention produced drawings rather like a ballet. In a farful emergency everybody goes into the right sort of place, and the most extraordinary shapes are made.'

In the rough and tumble of the daily theatre list, or the amphitheatre of professional and HNS politics, it is easy to overlook the beauty she describes. It springs from the values and skills of the poeple involvd and their ability to work as a team, respecting individual contributions and acknowledging how the whole they produce is greater than the sum of its parts. The values are embodied in words like dedication and commitment and altruism – which may sound a bit old-fashioned but are more needed than ever in the 21st century. They are also values which underlie this book and I hope you will read it absorb it, grow with it and enjoy it.

London 2000

Jane Salvage

REFERENCE

Hepworth B 1993 A pictorial autobiography. The Tate Gallery, London

Preface

The role of the theatre nurse has never been more secure or so volatile. These pages encapsulate the essence of perioperative nursing and reflect the true extent of the role. As one progresses through the pages, the ever-changing, multifaceted role of the perioperative nurse is unravelled – theatre nurse, recovery nurse, anaesthetic nurse, patient advocate, auditor, manager, quality assurer, advisor – it's all here.

Chapter 1, **Frameworks for care in perioperative nursing**, sets the scene and provides the opening words on the role of nurses and nursing in the perioperative setting. Written by a well-respected author, the chapter takes us through a range of care frameworks applicable to the care of a patient undergoing elective or emergency surgery.

Chapter 2, **Principles of safe practice in the perioperative environment**, provides an extensive overview of the key safety issues that all perioperative staff need to take into account. The perioperative environment is highly complex and practitioners are made aware of key legislation and the safety issues that must be addressed to ensure that patients are provided with competent and high-quality care.

Chapter 3, **Education for practice**, recognises the fact that perioperative nurses are lifelong learners and explains how all learners in the perioperative environment can be supported. The chapter also identifies the resources required for effective education in the perioperative setting and stresses the importance of self-directed learning and the need to appraise clinical practice.

Chapter 4, **Perioperative communication**, discusses one of the fundamental criteria which makes perioperative nursing so rewarding and so challenging. Working in a multidisciplinary team is not easy and is made more difficult when communications between professionals, and between nurse and patient, fail. This chapter outlines the essentials and gives guidance on how to improve communication in perioperative care.

Chapter 5, **Quality and quality assurance**, looks at what perioperative nurses do and how they could do it better; not by providing a blueprint for perioperative practice but by offering a way to measure the contribution of nursing care to the patient. Perioperative nursing is an art but it is essential that nurses evaluate their practice in order to ensure that what they do is the best possible. This chapter describes quality, the drive for quality, auditing and the concepts of best practice.

Chapter 6, **Perioperative risk management**, written by a renowned expert on managing health-care risk, emphasises the need to ensure that patient and staff safety is maintained through a proactive clinical risk management system. This chapter explains in detail the specific considerations that must be given to the perioperative environment to manage risks effectively and clarifies how this process relates to the principles of clinical governance.

Chapter 7, **Accountability and the law in perioperative care**, examines the issue of accountability and its complexities in perioperative care. The chapter explains how accountability works in practice and how all practitioners may be held to account for their actions or omissions.

Chapter 8, **Ethical issues in perioperative care**, explores the ethical issues that perioperative nurses face in their everyday practice. Drawing from key ethical theories and principles, this chapter discusses issues such as confidentiality, advocacy, consent and conscientious objection; all important ethical issues that require consideration and understanding by perioperative nurses.

Chapter 9, **Changing roles, changing titles in the perioperative environment**, looks at how the role of the perioperative nurse has changed over the last 20 years. This chapter takes the reader through the political and professional pressures to change and matches these pressures to the nursing response. This chapter is the key to understanding the change from theatre nurse to perioperative nurse.

Chapter 10, **Evidence-based practice in the perioperative environment**, highlights the importance of using evidence-based practice. This move away from traditional practice ensures that perioperative care is evidence-based. This is the root factor for providing excellent care.

Chapter 11, **Budgeting**, outlines that which is at the root of all evil: money. Financial restriction is a fact of life for all, yet an understanding of business planning and how budgets work can help to ensure that nurses are able to access available funds.

Chapter 12, **Information Technology**, is essential reading for today's perioperative nurse. The modern-day illiterates can read and write. What they cannot do is learn, unlearn and relearn new skills and knowledge. Information overload is a modern disease brought about by the proliferance of computer technology. A single edition of *The Times* holds more information than a 16th-century man would come across in a lifetime. This chapter outlines the information available today and how to use it effectively.

Chapter 13, **Recruitment and retention issues**, looks at an issue that must be top of every manager's agenda. In today's competitive world the challenge of recruitment and retention in the operating department threatens the existence of perioperative nursing, as we know it. This chapter examines recruitment and retention issues, describes their causes and suggests a strategy for addressing the problem. It touches on the factors inherent in the perioperative environment which can be used to enhance job excitement and influence the role.

Chapter 14, **Excellence in perioperative practice**, draws together all the principles of perioperative care and attempts to define perioperative excellence. Using real examples from perioperative practice, this chapter identifies how theoretical and practical learning combines with teamwork to create the conditions for developing excellence in perioperative practice.

The term 'perioperative' is an evolving one – its use still tends to change from one user to the next. In the context of this book, a perioperative nurse is a nurse who works in any area where surgery or anaesthesia takes place. The term 'perioperative practitioner' is used to denote any professional (for example nurse or operating department practitioner) involved in the care and support of the patient during surgery and anaesthesia. The term 'perioperative' encompasses anaesthetic, surgical and recovery skills and, in concept, places patient care and support at the centre of these roles. The 'surgical' and 'anaesthetic' teams describe the relevnt medical staff. The term 'theatre nurse' is occasionally used in deference to practitioners who still like to describe themselves as such.

Bournemouth and Edinburgh, 2000   Martin Hind   C Paul Wicker

Acknowledgements

No man is an island – no masterpiece is ever created single-handed. Martin Hind and Paul Wicker would like to thank their families, friends and colleagues for all their help and support during the production of this book.

Frameworks for care in perioperative nursing

Bernice J M West

INTRODUCTION

In the context of perioperative care, nurses tend to be biased towards action. In recent years, however, nurses in all contexts of care have been encouraged to ensure that their actions are evidence based and accountable. To do so, it is necessary to deploy an integrated framework for practice in the operating department. This chapter outlines a range of care frameworks which are applicable to the care of a patient undergoing elective or emergency surgery.

FRAMING PATIENT CARE

To effectively use a framework to guide perioperative nursing care, certain competencies are required. First, a sound **theoretical knowledge** is necessary so that nurses not only 'know how' to care but also they 'know why' care is being delivered in a particular way.

Second, **organisational skills** are required in order to coordinate nursing activities and in some contexts also the activities of other health professionals.

Third, **cognitive judgement skills** allow the nurse to perceive the need for care and actively provide that care in a sensitive way.

Finally, sophisticated **interpersonal skills** are required so that the chosen framework for care is understood by members of the perioperative health-care team and by patients. Without these skills and knowledge the perioperative nurse will have difficulties in using a nurse-led framework of care in the perioperative context.*

MODELS OF NURSING**

Nursing models can be defined as collections of ideas and concepts which describe in theoretical terms the major components of and external factors

---

* This chapter will not address these issues in detail. For further information, see Benner P 1984 From novice to expert: promoting excellence and career development in clinical nursing practice. Addison Wesley, Menlo Park, California. Schon D 1983 The reflective practitioner: how professionals think in action. Temple Smith, London.
** Parts of this section have been slightly modified from the original version in West BJM 1992 Theatre nursing technique and care. Baillière Tindall, London.

which affect nursing care. Models provide a framework around which nurses can plan patient care. There are many models of nursing. Existing conceptual models build upon one another and it is often cross-fertilisation of ideas from one model to another which results in enhanced practice.

In any practice setting, it is essential that the nurse selects an appropriate model to suit the clinical environment and meet the needs of patients. In perioperative nursing, there are two conceptual models which can be transferred easily into practice without having to reconstruct multidisciplinary approaches to health care. These are the self-care model (Orem 1980) and the activities of daily living model (Roper et al 1980). The Orem model works well with the practice of primary nursing in the context of day surgery. The Roper et al model is conceptually congruent with the current multidisciplinary approach to health-care organisation of integrated care pathways or managed clinical networks.

Self-care

This model was developed by Orem (1980). It is based on two types of self-care and the model sets out ways in which nurses can assess any self-care deficits in patients and plan nursing interventions accordingly. This model is particularly useful for theatre nurses involved in day surgery, where discharge planning and the emphasis on self-care are very important. Orem classifies self-care into two types.

The first type of self-care is called 'universal self-care'. This consists of the actions that human beings carry out and can be categorised as health maintenance activities.

- Maintenance of air, food and water. Each of these is essential to life, growth, development and the repair of body tissue.
- The process of excretion. As life continues, the human body processes food and oxygen and produces waste materials that need to be excreted.
- Maintenance of a balance between activity and rest. Certain levels of activity and rest are required for the human body to function well.
- Maintenance of a balance between solitude and social interaction. Normal human development requires periods of being alone and also periods of interaction with others.
- Prevention of hazards to human life and well-being. This involves the avoidance of conditions or situations that threaten or endanger the life of the individual.
- The maintenance of behaviour, health, well-being and lifestyle that are perceived to be within normal limits. Most individuals conform to what is considered to be socially and culturally acceptable.

The second type of self-care is termed 'health deviation self-care'. When a person undergoes changes in physical functioning or behaviour or ability to carry out activities of living, due to disease, injury or surgery, extra demands are made by that person. Therefore, when a loss of normal self-care ability takes place, the person can either make up the amount of self-care needed personally or else seek some kind of intervention. In the case of surgical patients, this intervention is usually nursing care, in which case the nurse may compensate wholly or partly for the self-care of the patient or educate and develop the patient to achieve full self-care.

Primary or named nursing*

Primary or named nursing is designed to assist with individualised patient care. The practice encompasses the philosophy of care which has been constructed for the clinical environment and a method of work organisation. A primary or named nursing approach to care enables the nurse to use whichever model of care best suits the patient and the environment. It provides the ideal vehicle for the nursing process, as it allows an individual nurse to assess, plan, implement and evaluate the care of a specific caseload of patients. Primary nurses are responsible and accountable for their own actions.

In addition to managing their own work, primary nurses also manage that of their associate nurses. Ideally, the primary nurse will work exclusively with a personal caseload of patients and has 24-hour responsibility for care. In consultation with the patient, the primary nurse plans and evaluates the care and, whilst on duty, delivers the planned care; when off duty, this planned care is delivered by the associate nurse. The associate nurse may add to the care plan and should discuss changes with the primary nurse at the earliest opportunity.

According to Manthey (1980), primary nursing is a method of organising nursing care which is based on four design elements.

1. Responsibility for the quality of nursing care
2. Care giver as care planner
3. Daily assignment by case
4. Direct channels of communication

The day surgery unit is the optimum environment for the practice of primary nursing in the context of perioperative nursing as the nurse will be able to incorporate the four design elements from the preassessment clinical phase through to discharge. To illustrate the applicability of this framework, each design element will be discussed briefly. The philosophy of care which has been used to inform the content is one based on Orem's self-care model.

Responsibility for the quality of nursing care Primary nurses are charged with responsibility to provide optimum care for the patient. In addition, they are also accountable for that care and would normally disclose this to the patient. So, for example, at a preadmission clinic, primary nurses would inform patients that they will be responsible for their nursing care whilst in the unit and for coordinating care services following discharge. In the day surgery unit, the ultimate process of postoperative

* In this chapter the terms 'primary nurse' and 'named nurse' will be used interchangeably.

recovery is transferred to the domiciliary context. For this reason, it is important that primary nurses view their responsibility from preadmission preparation of the patient through to the postoperative domiciliary period.

Care giver as care planner When possible, the primary nurse responsible for planning patient care also provides that care whilst on duty. In the context of day surgery, the primary nurse is aiming to promote well-being during the perioperative period. This requires that a plan of care is constructed with the patient covering the areas detailed in Table 1.1.

In day surgery, the primary nurse can plan this range of care at a preadmission clinic and ensure that aspects of the care are devolved to appropriate associate nurses. Ideally, the primary nurse should be available to oversee the key transitional phases of recovery for the postsurgical patient and be in a position to evaluate the effectiveness of the nursing decisions.

Daily assignment by case In the day surgery unit* it is imperative that:

- patients are appropriately selected for this type of intervention and that advanced anaesthetic techniques are used;
- the unit is adequately resourced;
- planned discharge criteria are in place.

Table 1.1 Care planning in day surgery

Care plan focus	Examples of content
1. Knowledge about the operative procedure	Perioperative care transfers; anaesthesia; operative procedure; postoperative monitoring; pain management; wound management
2. Signs and symptoms of recovery	Generalised pain; wound pain; referred pain; swelling; bruising; nausea; grogginess; clumsiness; mood changes; sleep disturbances; mobility; appetite; sensory impairment
3. The facilitation from dependence to independence	What the patient can do for themselves and what they will need help with in the short, medium and longer terms; the duration of help and the need to reorganise aspects of home life
4. Referral to other care agencies	Community services; emergency back-up; gaining access to hospital; support role of family and informal carers

* The organisation and management of day surgery units are outwith the remit of this chapter. For further information see the following:
Macpherson I, Hagen S 1992 Day surgery practice in Scotland. University of Aberdeen Health Services Research Unit Report No. 3. West BJM, Lyon MH 1995 Day surgery: a cheap option or challenge to care? British Journal of Theatre Nursing 5(1): 5–8.

The best way of facilitating this process is the use of a nurse-led preassessment clinic, where primary nurse and patient can be matched for the day of surgery.

Direct channels of communication   The primary nurse is the key person who receives and gives information about the patient. Such an approach facilitates continuity of care, enhances accountability, reduces confusion and promotes effective communication.

Primary nursing provides a useful framework for care in the day surgery unit where nursing roles are being developed and where the service is essentially nurse led. Increasingly, nurses are expanding their scope of professional practice to include work previously undertaken by medical staff. This is particularly evident in the context of day surgery where many clinics are nurse led (Laurenson 1995, West 1995, 1999). In these units nurses may be providing a 'one-stop shop' for patients. The use of primary nursing enhances the accountability of the nurse and provides a practice-based advocacy role for the nurse (Ersser & Tutton 1991).

Activities of living model

This model was developed in the United Kingdom by Roper, Logan & Tierney in 1980. They identified 12 activities of living common to all people.

1. Maintaining a safe environment
2. Communicating
3. Breathing
4. Eating and drinking
5. Eliminating
6. Personal cleansing and dressing
7. Controlling body temperature
8. Mobilising
9. Working and playing
10. Expressing sexuality
11. Sleeping
12. Dying

Each activity of living is complex and often interrelated to others in the list. This model of nursing is useful for planning care for the majority of adult surgical patients. It provides a framework for care to be planned along a continuum of independence. In addition the activities of living are understood by all health professionals working within the perioperative setting. This helps to ensure continuation of care practices when patients move through different environments, for example, from the surgical ward to the operating department to intensive care and back to the surgical ward.

Planning and managing care

Tables 1.2, 1.3 and 1.4 outline some common activity of living problems which may be experienced by a range of surgical patients during the preoperative, intraoperative and postoperative phases.

Table 1.2 Planning care in the preoperative phase

Activity of living	Patient problem
Communication	*Fear* related to potential outcome of surgery. For most patients an operation is a daunting event, full of fears about the outcome and success of the operation. The role of the nurse in giving information and reassurance is essential to the patient's psychological well-being.
Dying	*Anticipatory grieving* due to the loss of part of the body. Regardless of which part of the body is to be lost, an individual will experience some form of grieving. This grieving process is most pronounced in surgical patients about to undergo mutilating surgery, e.g. mastectomy, amputation of a limb, extensive bowel surgery. Recognition of this process of grieving and the giving of advice to patients and their families about the normal course of events are important parts of nursing care.
Eating and drinking	*Alteration in nutrition.* The process of fasting for surgery will necessarily alter the patient's nutritional status. Because in some cases this may exacerbate a previous chronic condition of malnourishment, it is essential that this is assessed and major deficits or imbalances addressed.
Maintaining a safe environment	*Potential fluid volume deficit.* The process of fasting for surgery will have altered the patient's electrolyte and fluid balance. Furthermore, because the nature of the proposed surgery may result in extensive fluid loss, preventive measures such as preoperative intravenous infusions may be commenced.
Sleeping	*Sleep pattern disturbance.* Research studies have shown that the majority of patients in hospital do not sleep well due to unfamiliar surroundings, anxiety about personal health and noise. For the surgical patient the night before an operation may be fraught. It is therefore necessary to support and inform the patient and where necessary administer a previously prescribed sedative or hypnotic.
Maintaining a safe environment	*Anticipatory anxiety* due to unfamiliar environment and impending surgery. This is most marked in the reception area of the operating department or the anaesthetic room. If the nurse can inform the patient in advance of what to expect and if the physical environment is made comfortable, then the patient's feelings of stress will be minimised.

Table 1.3 Planning care in the intraoperative phase

Activity of living	Patient problem
Breathing	*Potential alterations in respiratory function*, due to anaesthesia. This requires the nurse to be aware of normal limits and to monitor the patient's respirations appropriately.
Maintaining a safe environment	*Potential fluid volume deficit*, due to blood loss during surgery. This requires that an accurate record of blood loss during surgery be maintained and recorded. A protocol for maximum levels of blood loss is useful and a recognised regimen for replacement fluids is available.
Maintaining a safe environment	*Potential for injury*, due to decreased level of consciousness. This requires the nurse to assess, plan and record the positioning of the patient, the movement of an unconscious patient and the safety precautions to be used with specific equipment, e.g. electrosurgery.
Mobilising	*Potential decrease in cardiac output*, due to anaesthesia, decreased mobility and venous pooling. This requires the nurse to assess the patient for positioning and the most appropriate type of venous stimulation during surgery and to apply venous stimulation without causing damage to tissue.

Table 1.4 Planning care in the postoperative phase

Activity of living	Patient problem
Mobilising	*Pain* related to surgical incision. This requires the nurse to assess pain experiences objectively through monitoring and subjectively from patient's accounts and to act in accordance with medical prescriptions or nursing orders to alleviate pain and reduce restlessness.
Maintaining a safe environment	*Potential injury*, due to returning level of consciousness. This requires the nurse to assess the patient's consciousness level and to ensure that the immediate environment is safe and remains so.
Breathing	*Ineffective airway clearance*, due to retained secretions. This requires the nurse to assess the respiratory function of the patient, to take preventive actions as appropriate and to obtain medical assistance if necessary.
Maintaining a safe environment	*Sensory-perceptual alterations*, due to returning level of consciousness. These require that the nurse orientate the patient to time, place and event. Prior warning of the potential for postoperative confusion helps alleviate these problems.

By specifying patient problems as outlined in Tables 1.2, 1.3 and 1.4, the nurse can begin to set standards or clinical outcomes which can be evaluated or audited in order to determine the effectiveness of nursing actions or interventions.

EVIDENCE-BASED PRACTICE AND DECISION MAKING

The practice of nursing involves the planning of effective health outcomes in conjunction with the patient and other health professionals. This process involves the deployment of evidence to support judgements and a sophisticated approach to decision-making in clinical practice.

Evidence-based practice involves moving away from decision making based solely on opinion, past practice and precedence towards the inclusion of research and artistic evidence. It is an iterative process involving the assessment of fresh information and the evaluation of clinical action at successive stages. In the psychology of decision-making, this requires that the nurse begins to optimise the decision-making process. There is evidence to suggest that traditional 'minimal' nurses only obtained sufficient information to tackle the immediate clinical issue with which they were confronted (West 1992). This process of decision-making can be termed **satisficing** (West 1992) – as sufficient unto itself – but not optimal. The alternative approach to decision-making is **optimising**. This superior process occurs where the nurse has garnered optimal information and evidence from a variety of sources to improve all decision-making processes. Crucial to this mode is the nurse's ability to:

- portray a sophisticated use of clinical skills such as diagnosis, assessment and evaluation;
- deploy a wide range of knowledge bases;
- interact effectively with other professionals and patients;
- analyse and evaluate practice.

Making nursing assessments

The previous section has suggested that evidence-based practice is desirable in perioperative settings. This requires highly skilled nurses who can assess, make diagnoses and plan evidence-based interventions which allow for the evaluation of health outcomes.

The term 'nursing diagnosis' can be defined as the act of identifying and listing responses to actual or potential health problems or stressors. In the context of perioperative nursing, this definition is most useful as it works well within an integrated model which combines the values of self-care with the application of assessment techniques derived from activities of living. At the same time, it allows the delivery of nursing care to be organised according to the principles of primary or named nursing.

Nursing assessments and diagnoses provide the basis for selecting nursing interventions in order to achieve the health outcomes for which the nurse is accountable. Such diagnoses complement and enhance the care programmes instigated by other health professionals.

In order to make an informed nursing diagnosis, it is necessary to systematically collect information from the patient. Nursing is primarily concerned with the human response to actual or potential health problems whereas medicine is concerned with the identification and aetiology of a health problem. During a nursing history, information is elicited about individual responses to actual or potential health problems. This information, coupled with that of other professionals, provides the foundation for the nursing diagnoses and integrated planned interventions.

Throughout an episode of care the nurse who is practising in this integrated way will normally be expected to:

- review the reliability and validity of the information obtained;
- reflect on the information with regard to previous knowledge;
- plan effective health outcomes based on good practice and patient involvement;
- decide on optimum nursing interventions to enable the health outcomes to happen.

In this process of nursing subjective data are collected from the patient which cover the four key domains of health (West 1992).

1. *Somatological health:* care of the body and functional activities
2. *Social health:* relational well-being and involvement of others
3. *Psychological health:* emotional well-being and coping strategies
4. *Health maintenance activities:* actions regularly carried out by the individual and health professionals to optimise health and manage illnesses

In addition, objective data are gathered using a systems approach to the human body. Each of the major body systems is examined and measurements are taken as appropriate. By combining such approaches, immediate, short, medium and long-term health outcomes can be identified in accordance with planned nursing interventions and the health-care priorities of the patient.

The four domains of health and the associated subdomains within each may be used as the basis for a nursing assessment, planned interventions and for specifying health outcomes. In everyday life healthy individuals normally care for themselves within and across these four domains. When carrying out a thorough nursing assessment upon which to form nursing diagnoses and interventions, it is essential to establish the patient's normal self-care practices. A care plan can then be developed which optimises the patient's health status and level of independence and at the same time identifies realistic health outcomes.

Table 1.5 outlines the four key domains of health and their associated subdomains. In addition, examples of assessment queries to determine normal self-care practices are also provided.

Table 1.5 Nursing assessment process

Domain	Assessment queries to determine usual self-care practices
Somatological health	
Subdomains	
Elimination pattern	Description of usual bowel and urinary patterns
	Use of external aids
	Description of usual perspiration patterns
	Signs of itching
	Menstrual cycle
Activity and exercise patterns	Description of energy requirements for normal activities
	Usual type of exercise and range of activities
	Signs of breathlessness, chest pain, palpitations, stiffness, aching muscles and weakness
	Ability to carry out normal functional activities, e.g. feeding self
	Cooking
	Bathing and grooming
	Dressing
	Bed mobility
	General mobility
	Toileting
	Home maintenance activities
	Shopping
Nutrition	Typical daily food intake
	Use of supplements
	Typical daily fluid intake
	Weight change
	Appetite
	Discomfort associated with food
	Food preferences
	Food allergies
	Skin problems
	Healing potential
	Dental problems
Sleep and rest	Usual sleep pattern
	Usual sleep rituals
	Effect of sleep on preparedness for daily activities
Social health	
Subdomain	
Role and relationship patterns	Description of normal living arrangements
	Description of normal processes for resolving problems
	Significant others, feelings about illness
	Description of normal social encounters and activities
	Effects of current illness on normal social activities

Psychological health

Subdomains

Coping and stress management	Causes of tension
	What helps to alleviate tensions
	Recent life changes
	Usual problem-solving techniques
	Strategies for managing pain
Self-awareness	Normal self-description
	Effects of illness on self-description
Values and beliefs	General satisfaction with life
	Special health beliefs
	Special religious beliefs
	Any conflict between beliefs and health-care treatment
Cognitive patterns	Description of usual functioning of senses and memory
	Easiest way to learn things
	Normal communication patterns
	Understanding of present illness
	Understanding of treatments
	Description of usual sexual relations
	Effect of illness or treatments on sexuality

Health maintenance

Subdomain

Health perception	General state of health and reason for visit
	Identification of most important things done to keep healthy
	Current medication

By conducting such an assessment, the nurse will obtain a self-report account from patients about their health and the normal management strategies deployed. In addition, a series of physical examinations and measurements may also be undertaken to determine the normal functioning of the bodily systems as illustrated in Box 1.1.

A physical examination may also be carried out by means of inspection, percussion, auscultation and palpation. The information gained from these procedures can then be used alongside the assessments of other health professionals to plan health outcomes for the patient. These will be personalised yet also standardised according to nursing diagnoses. A comprehensive assessment and identification of diagnoses facilitate a holistic approach to determining socially meaningful health outcomes for surgical patients.

Box 1.1 Functional assessment

General state of health	Stature, speech, body movements, nutritional status
Vital signs	Blood pressure, pulse, respirations, temperature
Integument	Colour, lesions, scars, oedema, turgour, vascularity

INTEGRATED OPTIMAL CARE PLANNING*

In recent years there have been developments within the health service which require that nurses critically audit and evaluate the nature of their working practice. This has led to the setting of clinical standards focused on issues which combine structural aspects of care with the nursing process in order to achieve specific care outcomes. In the past nursing standards have been uniprofessional but clinical governance now allows nursing the opportunity to construct clinical standards which are relevant to other disciplines and indeed may form the basis of integrated care pathways.

The operational framework for nurses is called **integrated optimal care planning**. This approach to nursing is idealistic yet pragmatic, calling for both personal commitment and interprofessional coordination. In knowledge terms, it requires a sound information base and extensive problem-solving skills. To illustrate the processes involved in producing such integrated optimal care plans, with identified health outcomes, it is necessary to address both the diagnostic aspects and the interventionist nature of planned nursing care in perioperative settings.

Integrated optimal care plans

Integrated optimal care plans provide documentary evidence of the range of care being given to any one patient by the full multidisciplinary team. Using the information obtained from the assessments and other literature, outcomes are agreed with the patient. Then, by means of a multidisciplinary and patient-centred conference, interventions can be planned. Interventions will be based upon sound rationales, intuition, creativity, availability of resources and, when patients are able, their preferences.

Nursing interventions can be considered as any direct action performed, on behalf of a patient, by a nurse or appropriately designated others. Actions may be initiated by the nurse following the identification of a nursing diagnosis, by physician-initiated treatments or by the identification of essential daily activities that the patient cannot perform independently.

In planning effective health care, it is the integration of all health professional activities that leads to successful health outcomes. Thus, it is not sufficient for the care plans to be uniprofessional; optimal care plans are integrated and multiprofessional. Integrated clinical practice provides the means of directing the health-care team in daily activities to optimise patient health and well-being. It includes a care plan which covers the pre-hospitalisation, hospitalisation and posthospitalisation phases. Patient health outcomes and clinical effectiveness are enhanced as the activities of each professional group in each stage of the process are made explicit.

---

* This section has been adapted from the original by West B J M, Lyon M H 1999 Measuring health outcomes. In: Manley K, Bellman L (eds) Perioperative nursing. Churchill Livingstone, London.

An integrated optimal care plan outlines the clinical practice and treatment requirements for a patient at specified times throughout the period of ill health or dependency. The benefits of such an approach to care planning are:

- improved interprofessional communication;
- constant review and development of care practices;
- reduction in duplication of documentation by the various health professionals;
- discharge planning is made evident from the time of admission to hospital;
- clinical audit data are readily available;
- an evidence-based culture of care is promoted.

To introduce such an approach to health-care planning requires considerable effort from all disciplines involved. The current focus on clinical governance may provide the impetus for a more collective approach to management of acute care. Box 1.2 shows how an integrated care plan could be laid out.

Box 1.2   Integrated optimal care plan

		Time			
Focus of care	*Preadmission clinic*	*Day 1*	*Day 2*	*Day 3*	*Day 4*
Assessments					
Tests/Results					
Surgery					
Medications					
Activities of living					
1. Maintaining a safe environment					
2. Communicating					
3. Breathing					
4. Eating and drinking					
5. Eliminating					
6. Personal cleansing and dressing					
7. Controlling body temperature					
8. Mobilising					
9. Working and playing					
10. Expressing sexuality					
11. Sleeping					
12. Dying					
Discharge plans					

The multidisciplinary team carries out the construction of an integrated care plan. In the perioperative setting, this team may comprise:

- primary or named nurse;
- anaesthetist;
- surgeon;
- physiotherapist.

In the planning phase the team will consider:

- the patient health outcomes;
- the optimum way of achieving the desired outcomes;
- who in the team is accountable for ensuring that these outcomes are achieved;
- the structure and phasing of care.

Total hip replacement

This section will provide examples of an integrated care plan covering a particular surgical intervention. The area selected is typical of surgery performed in most surgical units.

Total hip replacement is an important and seminal advancement in reconstructive surgery. It has provided significant relief of pain and improved physical functioning for patients with arthritis. Hip replacement is widely used in the treatment of osteoarthritis and rheumatic arthritis as well as for hip fractures.

The nursing care of the patient undergoing a total hip replacement must begin with education and the setting of realistic goals. The preparation for surgery, duration of hospital stay and expected postoperative events must each be discussed with the patient and others in order that realistic and effective health outcomes can be identified. The long-term health benefits to the patient are considerably greater than the costs of carrying out the surgery.

To illustrate the process, nursing diagnoses have been identified (Box 1.3). From these an integrated care plan can be developed in conjunction with other health professionals.

It is only by integrating care planning across the disciplines and across the care environments that these health outcomes can be achieved (Box 1.4).

ORGANISATIONAL REQUIREMENTS

Health and illness are complex concepts which have their bases in subjective experiences. In helping a patient achieve a state of health, the nurse must take into consideration the multiple factors involved; consequently it is suggested that health outcomes must be equally refined. Health is a dynamic state which reflects an equilibrium across the four domains of health (West 1992) which were discussed previously. Each patient can be

---

Box 1.3   Examples of nursing diagnoses

---

*Specific postsurgical nursing diagnoses: total hip replacement**
1. Impaired physical mobility related to pain, stiffness and surgical procedure.
2. Reluctance, unwillingness or inability to participate in physical rehabilitation.
3. Expressed fear of walking and/or moving.
4. Self-care deficits due to restrictions imposed by surgery.
5. Expressed fear of performing normal daily routines.

1. Risk of infection related to exposure of joint during surgery.
2. Risk of infection due to environmental pathogens.
3. Risk of infection due to ineffective prophylaxis.

1. Risk of personal injury related to pain, weakness, fatigue, orthostatic hypotension.
2. Risk of personal injury related to use of ambulatory aids.

1. Risk of ineffective management of care regimen due to lack of knowledge.
2. Risk of ineffective personal coping strategies due to unrealistic expectations.
3. Risk of ineffective personal coping strategies due to inadequate support mechanisms.

Specific collaborative diagnoses
1. Risk of peripheral neurovascular dysfunction.
2. Risk of dislocation of prosthesis due to improper movement and/or infection.
3. Risk of thrombophlebitis due to surgery and immobilisation.

---

* These data first appeared in West B J M, Lyon M H 1999 Measuring health outcomes. In Manley K, Bellman L (eds) Perioperative nursing. Churchill Livingstone, London.

Box 1.4   Examples of health outcomes to be achieved prior to discharge

---

- Patients have a decrease in or absence of pain as measured by a pain assessment tool and expressed satisfaction of patient.
- Patients have sufficient muscle strength to continue an activity programme designed to optimise their walking gait as measured by clinical indicators of muscle strength devised by physiotherapist.
- Patients' mobility is restored and they can use walking aids optimally as measured by a staged activity-programmed, self-assessment process and absence of postoperative complications, e.g. flexion contracture of the hip.
- Patients have healthy skin as measured by pressure area and wound assessment tools used by the primary nurse.
- Patients are free from infection as measured by temperature, photographs of wound site.
- Patients have a personal plan for managing care at home as documented by primary nurse and shared with community nurse and patient with specified goals.
- Patients are confident of their recovery process as measured by a self-report scale covering well-being and anxiety.

assessed on these domains and commonalties based on illness or diagnostic groups can be discerned. From this, aspects of perioperative nursing care can be standardised in part and integrated and refined health outcomes can be specified. However, to enhance the clinical practice of the nurse in each of the care environments, the personalised and individuated nature of patient need must also be included to ensure a high quality of health care for all patients.

In perioperative care settings, it is important that the professional can deliver expert care to the patient. It would be naive to assume that a nurse in a surgical setting has limitless time to make optimal decisions or limitless resources to conduct sophisticated research. Consequently, if a provider of health services truly wishes to offer health care of the highest human and technical quality in accordance with the current demands of clinical governance, then investment is necessary. This must include investment in:

- the education and training of health professionals and other health-care workers;
- the deployment of sufficient professionals and other health-care workers;
- research;
- the education of patients about treatment and care options.

Evidence-based practice will influence many aspects of nursing care in perioperative settings and such an approach will result in patients receiving optimum care. Indeed, if this integrated model of clinical decision making is endorsed and seriously upheld by clinicians, health service managers and politicians, then there will be many beneficial effects on the health of the workforce and their patients.

REFERENCES

Ersser S, Tutton E 1991 Primary nursing in perspective. Scutari, London

Laurenson S 1995 Health service developments and the scope of professional nursing practice: a survey of clinical role developments in NHS Trusts in Scotland. HMSO, Edinburgh.

Manthey M 1980 The practice of primary nursing. Blackwell, Boston

Orem D 1980 Nursing concepts of practice. McGraw Hill, New York

Roper N, Logan W, Tierney A 1980 The elements of nursing. Churchill Livingstone. Edinburgh

West B J M 1992 Nurses' perceptions in the nursing process: a study of two cardiothoracic units. PhD thesis, University of Edinburgh

West B J M 1995 Health service developments and the scope of professional nursing practice: a review of pertinent literature. HMSO, Edinburgh

West B J M 1999 Role development in nursing and midwifery – so where are we now? A review of research literature. HMSO, Edinburgh

Principles of safe practice in the perioperative environment

2

Sheila Turner   Paul Wicker
Martin Hind

INTRODUCTION

The perioperative environment is possibly the most hazardous of all clinical environments for patient and staff alike. The combination of rapid client throughput and the quantities of noxious materials employed in surgical intervention is a potential minefield. Perioperative practitioners do not, however, have to negotiate this minefield daily, providing they pay scrupulous attention to their management of the perioperative environment and comply with legislation.

It might be amusing to assume that 'rules are made to be broken' and most of us take this attitude at some time in our professional lives but ignorance of the law is no defence when things go wrong.

This chapter includes consideration of legislation relevant to the perioperative environment and explores key safety issues in perioperative care.

Duty of care

According to Dimond (1995), 'Duty of care can be said to exist if one can see that one's actions are reasonably likely to cause harm to another person'.

As nurses owe a 'duty of care' to their patients, so their employers (NHS trusts, etc.) owe them a 'duty of care' in ensuring a safe working environment. Duty of care is regulated by civil (as opposed to criminal) law (see Chapter 7). Judicial rulings are based upon case law, i.e. previous decisions made in similar cases. There is an order of precedence, at the top of which is the House of Lords whose decision is binding upon all other courts in the United Kingdom. The House of Lords can only be overruled by the European Court of Justice. As will become evident, European law has an increasing influence upon UK nursing practice.

The nurse's role

The nurse's role is summarised in *Exercising accountability* (UKCC 1989) and the *Code of professional conduct* (UKCC 1992) in terms of patient safety, security and the need for risk assessment.

The nurse must always promote and safeguard the interests and well-being of the patient and ensure that no action or omission in her area of responsibility is detrimental to the patient. (UKCC 1992)

There is an onus upon nurses to keep up to date with current practice/legislation, etc. so that they are best prepared to manage any situation. When things go wrong, although nurses bear the burden of responsibility, they cannot necessarily be blamed. The fact that many employers accept vicarious liability for their professional staff offers some security. However, the individual must acknowledge responsibility if working beyond what might be considered appropriate for their role.

The 1995 case of a UK theatre sister who performed an appendicectomy, practising beyond what is accepted for the role of theatre sister, has made perioperative practitioners examine the scope of their practice, questioning how far their roles have expanded; also, whether employers recognise their evolving role, without which the professional would be personally liable for any mistakes they might make.

This reinforces the need for nurses to be informed about legislation and potential litigation. One significant area of legislation places a clear responsibility upon both employer and employee: the Heath and Safety at Work Act 1974.

The nurse must have regard to the environment and its physical, psychological and social effects on the patient and to the adequacy of resources and inform appropriate authorities of any circumstance which could place the patient at risk or which militate against safe standards of practice. (UKCC 1989)

Health and safety is everybody's responsibility.

HEALTH AND SAFETY AT WORK LEGISLATION

It shall be the duty of every employee, while at work, to take reasonable care for the health and safety of himself and of the other persons who may be affected by his actions and omissions. (Health and Safety at Work Act 1974)

Amazingly, the NHS was slow to respond to this new legislation. The NHS and Community Care Act 1990 resulted in the loss of Crown immunity and the need to comply fully with all aspects of the law. The Health and Safety at Work Act can be summarised thus:

- Protecting the health, safety and welfare of the 'worker'.
- Protecting users, consumers and visitors from any hazards associated with the workplace and the workforce.
- Controlling the storage, handling and use of hazardous materials.

The employer has an obligation to the employee. As far as is reasonable, the employer must provide appropriate safe access and egress to and from the working environment; this includes lighting and signing, fire exits, etc. The workplace itself must be suitable for the nature of the work; for example, if the floor is going to be made wet as a result of the work it needs to have adequate drainage, possibly a non-slip surface, personnel might need protective footwear, the area will require frequent cleaning to minimise the risk of falls. What happens in your scrub area? In many, the floor is a real hazard.

The workplace must be adequately illuminated, ventilated and heated for optimum working conditions.

The employer must provide adequate facilities to move, manipulate and manage equipment and materials; this includes the provision of adequate storage facilities.

The workforce must be properly informed about their role and should receive tuition in the function and use of new equipment or procedures. Any lack of clarity may lead to errors which could result in accidental injury; something wholly preventable may result in the employee responsible and their employer being called to account.

The employer is required to provide a written health and safety policy statement, the contents of which have to be regularly reviewed, updated and circulated to all employees. Regular health and safety audits highlight good practice, as well as areas of concern.

The Act requires the appointment of trades union health and safety representatives whose role is to negotiate with employer and employees on issues related to health and safety.

It is necessary to employ risk assessment and management strategies to reduce all identified risks to an acceptable level. The Health and Safety at Work Act also imposes responsibility on the manufacturers of equipment and materials so that:

- they are safely assembled/manufactured;
- they have been tested;
- users have received appropriate training;
- where there may be a hazard, it is clearly indicated to the user;
- adequate research has been completed to ensure that the item is safe to use;
- where an item has to be installed, the manufacturer oversees installation.

Employees have considerable responsibility.

- To carry out their duties as identified by their employer.
- To protect themselves and others who may be affected by what they are doing.
- They must not mishandle or abuse any equipment which is provided for their use, particularly as defective equipment may endanger themselves, a subsequent user or even the client of their service.

An appropriate example to consider might be the anecdotal evidence that some practitioners bend needles before cannulating patients; it is suggested that some even snap off the hub before cannulating babies, allowing blood to trickle freely from the broken end into a specimen container.

Manufacturers rightly refuse to accept any responsibility for this abuse of their product.

A patient can use the Consumer Protection Act 1987 if defective equipment has injured them. Anyone making a claim for compensation has to prove that the device that is claimed to have harmed them was being used for the purpose stipulated by its manufacturers. In the example of practitioners altering devices/equipment, the practitioner becomes personally liable should harm result.

There must be a mechanism whereby employees can feedback to management their concerns about hazardous situations or practice. They must feel confident that they will not be subject to harassment or censure for their 'whistleblowing'.

The Health and Safety Commission, Executive and Inspectorate have been established to ensure that health and safety regulations are enforced by providing practical guidance and codes of practice and ultimately imposing sanctions on those organisations who do not conform to the legislation. The Inspectorate can serve improvement and prohibition notices, closing premises they consider unsafe. They can seize items, materials or machinery considered to be an immediate danger and destroy them. Civil action is the result of failure to comply with health and safety legislation.

Because, according to Health and Safety Executive statistics, 400+ people die at work in the UK each year and over 12 000+ suffer major injuries, employers must:

- identify health hazards;
- develop methods to minimise or prevent hazards;
- carry out health screening and biological monitoring;
- provide health education, counselling and rehabilitation;
- train and supervise first-aiders;
- ensure the thorough completion of documentation;
- seek advice, when necessary.

Physical injury is not the only problem; stress is becoming a significant issue to health and safety at work. Stress is not caused directly by situations but how individuals respond mentally to them. There is a clear physiological link as sufferers prepare for 'fight or flight' in reaction to 'threats'. Repeated initiation of this response places pressure on both the immune and cardiovascular systems. In some individuals just thinking about a situation can provoke this response. Initially a sufferer from stress might display many symptoms of being 'run down', frequent coughs and colds, etc., before more serious symptoms manifest.

Employees have gained compensation where the effects of stress have prevented them from doing their job. As Seymour (1995) notes, in 1994 John Walker successfully sued his employer, Northumberland County Council, for causing his second nervous breakdown due to extreme workload and lack of support. And in 1995 Dr Chris Johnstone settled out of court, gaining £5000 compensation from Camden and Islington Health Authority for an excessive workload, which he maintained had led him to become suicidally depressed.

The Health and Safety at Work Act remains a powerful piece of legislation, strengthened by:

- Control of Substances Hazardous to Health (COSHH) 1988;
- COSHH revision re exposure to medical gases, volatile agents and vapours 1994;
- The 'six-pack' – six regulations which have been adopted as a result of European directives; these clarify and strengthen the original legislation. The 'six-pack' comprises:
  1. Management of Health and Safety at Work Regulations 1992
  2. Workplace Health, Safety and Welfare Regulations 1992
  3. The Provision and Use of Work Equipment Regulations 1992
  4. The Personal Protective Equipment at Work Regulations 1992
  5. The Display Screen Equipment Regulations 1992
  6. Manual Handling Operations Regulations 1992.

Control of Substances Hazardous to Health 1988 and Occupational Exposure Standards 1994

Originally all substances which might be classified as 'very toxic, toxic, harmful, corrosive or irritant' were included in the Classification, Packaging and Labelling Regulations 1984. Now, using the same descriptors of materials potentially hazardous to health plus those materials having recognised maximum exposure limits (MEL) or occupational exposure standards (OES), microorganisms hazardous to health and dust are all managed under the umbrella of COSHH. The requirements of COSHH are:

- audit of environment and personnel;
- the use of risk assessment and management;
- control of risks that cannot be eliminated;
- personnel to be informed of the hazards to their health;
- use of appropriate facilities, e.g. fume cabinets;
- training personnel in the safest methods of storage, handling and use of hazardous materials;
- appropriate policies and procedures;
- provision of protective clothing/equipment.

An initial COSHH assessment should have identified:

- any hazardous materials and whether they could be eliminated from use;
- an action plan for the improved management of all materials of concern.

Audit should be an ongoing process; there must be a regular review of the COSHH assessment to ensure that all concerned are protected from hazards.

Materials of concern to the perioperative practitioner include:

- inhalational anaesthesia;
- glutaraldehyde and formaldehyde;
- methyl methacrylate (cement);
- pathogenic microorganisms, e.g. Tuberculosis bacillus (TB), methicillin-resistant *Staphylococcus aureus* (MRSA) and hepatitis C – sometimes inaccurately described as airborne (TB and MRSA) and bloodborne (hepatitis C);
- dusts – the accumulation of dust as a vector of infection or specific dusts, e.g. wood or plaster of Paris;
- powerful disinfectants, e.g. hypochlorite solutions;
- latex;
- radiation;
- lasers.

MEL are a maximum value of exposure to a hazardous material. OES give a value to the limit of exposure which must not be exceeded and are expressed as concentrations in air parts per million (ppm) (see Table 2.1).

Where materials hazardous to health are regularly employed, all personnel involved need health surveillance to ensure that their health is not adversely affected. This is very important as methods to measure an individual's exposure to anaesthetic gases (for example) are inadequate. Each agent needs a specific monitoring device and the measurement process is lengthy and often expensive. Even where waste gas scavenging is operational, personnel who are obliged to, for example, fill vaporisers without provision of fume cabinets are at risk of exposure to high concentrations of the agents. In the recovery room, where scavenging is almost impossible to achieve, the nurses are frequently exposed to significant concentrations of anaesthetic agents as recovering patients breathe in and out.

A number of materials in the operating department could be the 'villains' in the acquisition of occupational asthma – there are currently 200 known 'sensitisers' across all occupations in the UK. The Health and Safety Executive estimates that there were over 1000 new cases of occupational asthma identified in 1992. It is difficult to determine how many cases are work related as the incidence of asthma is increasing generally. One clear

Table 2.1 Occupational exposure standards for glutaraldehyde, ethylene oxide and anaesthetic gases

Substance	8-hour exposure limit
Nitrous oxide	100 ppm
Enflurane	20 ppm
Halothane	10 ppm
Isoflurane	50 ppm
Glutaraldehyde	0.2 ppm
Ethylene oxide	0.5 ppm

indicator is that sufferers improve when they are away from work, the implication being that something at work is triggering the asthma attacks.

The aim of health surveillance is to identify personnel at risk and to define a baseline set of data which is used in comparison with subsequent measurements made annually (or as frequently as required by occupational health). So the surveillance should include vital signs, lung function and skin assessment because the incidence of contact and allergic dermatitis (and latex allergy) is also on the increase. This forms a vital part of risk assessment, allowing employers to acknowledge and manage risks before they cause ill health, to minimise identified health risks and to assess the efficiency of the interventions.

Glutaraldehyde (see also Sterilisation techniques, p. 31)

Glutaraldehyde poses a great risk to health. Even when exposed to low airborne concentrations, nurses have developed rhinitis, runny eyes and a wheezy chest. It is vital that personnel observe recommendations involving the (non) handling of glutaraldehyde: adequate ventilation, partial enclosure with local exhaust ventilation, the use of nitrile gloves, wearing goggles, gowns and aprons to minimise skin contact. COSHH stipulates that products like glutaraldehyde only be used where there is no suitable alternative. At present other products surpass glutaraldehyde in antimicrobial activity but are more toxic, more damaging to instruments or more expensive.

There is a need to exercise vigilance and diligence in the management of glutaraldehyde. Hutt (1994) details the problems associated with glutaraldehyde as 'short-term exposure, skin exposure and lengthy exposure'.

- Short-term exposure can lead to: respiratory irritation, bronchial constriction, occupational asthma, watering eyes and facial dermatitis.
- Skin exposure can lead to: contact eczema, contact dermatitis, allergic dermatitis, nausea, headaches, dizziness and nervous tremor.
- Lengthy exposure can lead to: nausea and gastrointestinal symptoms, jaundice, circulatory problems, brain changes, mood swings, irritability, loss of judgement and depressed immune response.

Unfortunately, some nurses seem unable to accept that health and safety at work is a necessity, not a luxury. Too often excuses made for poor practice or working conditions include 'I did it to save time', 'I knew it wasn't right but ...'. This is an extremely short-sighted stance as work-injured nurses are hardly able to care for their patients when on protracted sick leave. Their sickness just increases the pressure on colleagues who have to cope in their absence.

A blame culture is very evident in the NHS and work-injured nurses seem reluctant to report the cause of their ill health for fear that they themselves will be blamed or, worse, that they will be unable to continue with their career.

MANUAL HANDLING

The literature suggests that one in four nurses has had time off due to a back injury sustained at work. The Health and Safety Executive (1991) identified that some 70% of work-related accidents involved manual handling (of people) and almost half the incidents resulted in back injury. Nationally, back pain is the greatest single cause identified for days lost to sickness. Barker et al (1994) estimate that 1.3 million working days are lost annually, in the NHS alone, because of back pain. Snell (1995) states that 80 000 nurses annually suffer back injury, 3600 of whom suffer disabling injury which results in their permanent loss to the profession. Prevention, as there is no 'cure', must be the aim for all practitioners.

Manual handling is defined by the Health and Safety Executive as: 'Any transporting or supporting of a load including the lifting, putting down, pushing, pulling, carrying or moving thereof by hand or bodily force' (Manual Handling Operations Regulations 1992). The Manual Handling Operations Regulations 1992 are enforced under the Health and Safety at Work Act, in response to European directives. They place an onus upon the employer to:

- assess the risk to the health and safety of employees;
- avoid hazardous manual handling operations;
- reduce the risk of injury by employing appropriate manual handling techniques.

The regulations require employees to:

- make use of equipment supplied for its proper purpose;
- accept training in the use of the equipment;
- adhere to policies and procedures in respect of manual handling.

The National Back Pain Association and the RCN (1997) have made specific recommendations for manual handling processes in the operating theatre. These can be summarised as follows.

- The need for all personnel, including medical staff, to be trained in manual handling techniques.
- Safe patient transfer onto the operating table, the easiest being lateral transfer with a rigid board, which can be cleaned immediately after use.
- The need for a policy statement on the management of larger clients who cannot be transferred using the lateral slide technique.
- Storage of heavy instrument trays at waist height.
- Distribution of instrument weight so that no single tray is too heavy for an individual to lift.
- Use of appropriate devices to minimise the lifting and movement of heavy equipment.
- Rolling patients rather than lifting them into a lateral position, using the sheet beneath them.

- Use of devices, rather than human team members, to support the limbs of anaesthetised patients; often the anaesthetic assistant has to elevate limbs for a considerable length of time during skin preparation and draping.
- Planning patient movement, accounting for the 'extras' that might accompany the patient to recovery, e.g. monitoring, catheters, etc.
- Recovering patients postoperatively on a height-adjustable trolley or bed; ideally transferring the patient to their own bed as quickly as is practicable.
- As torso, head and arms comprise 60% of body weight, elevating patients into a sitting position is best undertaken when the patients can move themselves.
- Patients who are too heavy to manoeuvre in this way should be nursed on a bed with a head section that can be easily elevated.

To minimise patient movement, many units allow patients into the operating department on their own bed, transferring them back onto the bed as soon as is practicable after surgery.

The literature indicates the need to employ an ergonomic approach to manual handling. So what are ergonomics? McFarlane (1995) defines ergonomics as 'the practical and scientific study of people in relation to their working environment.' There is the suggestion that ergonomics is related not only to the worker and the environment but also to the efficiency with which tasks are completed, the use of aids and methods which minimise the strain on the nursing staff as they plan to move or adjust the position of their patients. Before every manual handling procedure, the 'team' involved effectively undertake a risk assessment and choose the method best suited to minimise the identified risk. There is an emphasis upon teamwork and cooperation; agreement is achieved between all parties as to why, how and when patient movement and positioning will take place.

Thus the principles of manual handling might be outlined as follows.

1. Employ a 'no lifting' policy.
2. Assess the risks associated with the planned manoeuvre.
3. Consider the patient: can he assist the nurses?
4. Select appropriate aids.
5. Inform patient and colleagues of chosen method.
6. Gather together everything necessary.
7. Select an appropriate position and posture.
8. Remain as close to the patient as possible.
9. Exercise control by determining who does 'what' and 'when', e.g. 'ready, steady, slide!' when moving a patient from trolley to bed in the recovery room.

Many back injuries result from nurses responding to emergencies; for example, trying to stop patients from falling. All nurses must have regular refresher training on manual handling; their day-to-day patient management must be 'back friendly' and their response to emergencies should involve more caution and concern for their backs. So, when an emergency situation does arise, nurses are able to stop momentarily, assess the risks and select the best method to manage whatever problem confronts them.

WASTE MANAGEMENT AND DISPOSAL

The Environment Protection Act (1990) imposes a 'duty of care' on all responsible for waste disposal; this includes the organisations generating the waste. There is also a criminal liability on the waste disposal organisations. Apart from aesthetic considerations, it is wholly unacceptable that clinical waste be dumped on public landfill sites. Clinical waste might contain human tissue, body fluids, products contaminated from contact with human tissue and fluids, drug containers, administration devices, etc. This is why COSHH applies to clinical waste management. Clinical waste is best managed by incineration.

Most organisations have adopted a scheme of colour coding for waste disposal bags and containers.

- Yellow – clinical waste for disposal that requires incineration.
- Black – household waste, generated by offices and kitchens.
- Clear – sealed bags for the return of instruments to sterile services for cleaning, sterilisation or recycling.
- Aerosols and glass are a significant risk and have to be separately bagged; aerosols would explode upon incineration (possible when stored in a hot environment).

Waste bags should not be filled so full that they cannot easily be sealed with a knot. All bags of waste must be labelled, to indicate where they came from and when. In the operating department this can be particularly important: should towel clips or small instruments go missing, the waste can be retrieved and searched (with extreme caution, by gloved personnel) before any more dramatic action is taken, though it must be emphasised that good practice should negate this activity.

Waste should be collected promptly and removed to a secure container whilst awaiting incineration. The containers in which bags of waste are stored must be lockable and must have an easy-to-clean interior. Likewise, areas designated for waste management must be accessible for cleaning without posing a threat to the cleaners. If, for example, some noxious volatile liquid had been dumped in a waste disposal bag and the bag had been placed in an airtight room, the next person entering the room might be exposed to an unacceptable quantity of fumes. Consideration for others should be a key word in waste management.

Any spillages from bags of waste must be immediately cleaned up using an appropriate method. This is to minimise any slips and falls as well as to minimise exposure to potentially pathogenic material. According to local policy, small spills of blood are managed with hypochlorite granules, which can be dusted up and returned to the waste bag. Larger spills are managed with an equal volume of neat sodium hypochlorite solution which is mopped up. The bag should be resealed or the contents rebagged. It cannot go unremarked that mops and cleaning devices themselves pose a real threat to health. In the operating department, ideally, disposable mopheads should be used and then discarded; where old-style mops and buckets are in use the mopheads must be autoclaved regularly. Many areas still have festering brews sitting in their disposal rooms and quite often no one knows when the bucket was last cleaned out and fresh hot soapy water installed. In fact, mop and bucket should be stored dry when not in use.

All staff dealing with waste material must have access to handwashing facilities and are expected to wash their hands frequently, particularly if also involved in patient contact. Nurses seem unaware of how little they wash their hands between procedures, apparently immune to the hazardous effects of the materials they handle. Nurses might be more tolerant of unpleasant smells and the sight of damaged human tissue but all are at equal risk from the very real hazards of waste disposal.

The literature indicates that, with good practice, double bagging of waste is unnecessary, as is the labelling of material an 'infection hazard' because all material should be treated with equal caution. There is no excuse for sharps being found in waste disposal bags. If they are and the practitioner responsible can be traced, they might be deemed personally liable if someone handling the waste subsequently suffers a needlestick injury.

There should be adequate provision of sharps boxes so that practitioners are not tempted to put used sharps devices to one side. The priority in sharps management is the appropriate disposal of the sharp device. During a surgical procedure, 'sharps' are retained on the instrument trolley. Blades are only mounted onto or removed from blade handles with forceps, never by gloved hand alone. Needles are retained on a sticky pad or some other tool, so that they can be seen and easily counted by scrub and circulating nurse, prior to disposal in a sharps container by the scrub nurse. Sharps containers, like clinical waste disposal bags, are yellow. They are rigid plastic and must conform to BS 7320 which requires:

- instructions for container assembly;
- the presence of a handle;
- a device to close the container securely;
- that the container is leakproof and perforation proof and cannot be easily damaged;
- a fill-to-line indicator (everybody always discards their sharps container when only three-quarters full, don't they?);
- 'danger contaminated sharps' and 'destroy by incineration' labelling;
- the name of the manufacturer.

All these requirements are designed to offer optimum protection to 'those at the sharp end'.

The most dangerous time in sharps management is sharps disposal. The risk associated with poor technique or non-adherence to the guidelines is that someone, not necessarily the user of the sharp item, may suffer a traumatic injury. If the device is contaminated with patient blood or body fluids the injured individual may be exposed to any number of disease-causing organisms. The psychological trauma alone can be damaging: the antiviral treatment now offered where the donor of blood/body fluid is known to be HIV positive can be unpleasant for the recipient.

Case study 2.1

In 1998 an unnamed doctor won substantial damages (£500 000) for a needle-stick injury (Daily Mail 1998). She suffered no physical harm as a result of the injury but the psychological effects caused her to become fearful of work; eventually she became a prisoner in her own home. Many people complained about the amount she was awarded but the court decided that she needed to be fairly compensated for her lost career.

The used needle which injured the doctor was left, unsheathed, on the drug trolley. There was an obvious failure to comply with waste disposal policy: the needle should have been discarded in a sharps box immediately after use. Some organisations advocate taking the sharps box to the bedside so that disposal is immediate.

In practice, there are situations where nurses become distracted – an emergency, for example – but all practitioners should be aware of the risks that needlestick injuries present. What are the risks? Fifteen years ago it was the human immunodeficiency virus (HIV), a newly emerging and frightening virus. Now practitioners seem almost blasé about HIV, most have been immunised against hepatitis B and the major concern is hepatitis C. Hepatitis C is difficult to detect. Currently, it is most often acquired through blood transfusion. According to Domin (1995), once infected, 60% will develop chronic liver disease; of those, 20% will demonstrate chronic hepatitis over the course of the disease. A number of people infected with hepatitis C will develop hepatoma (liver cancer), a truly frightening prospect for a preventable incident. Because unsheathed hollow needles are the major 'vectors' in needlestick injury, a number of manufacturers have developed retractable (self-sheathing) needles to minimise the risk.

ASEPSIS

'Clean' implies 'without obvious contamination or soiling'. Thus, microorganisms might be lurking, invisible to the naked eye. This might be acceptable when talking about cutlery: even if contaminants are present on the surface of knives and forks, gastrointestinal pH should destroy them. However, the 'knives and forks' of surgery need to be more than just clean. At surgery, tissue which is sterile and closed is incised and exposed to the environment.

Any contaminants introduced at this time might cause devastating infections: at least, delaying wound healing; at worst, resulting in death. So surgical instruments need to be sterile – totally free of contaminants, living organisms, bacterial or fungal spores. Spores are the most resistant forms of life, surviving extremes of heat, cold, hydration and desiccation.

Degrees of cleanliness are recognised and accepted for specific procedures.

• *Cleaning* – a process which removes all debris and the material on which microorganisms exist. Achieved with soaps or detergents and hot water. All surgical instruments must be thoroughly cleaned according to local policy and dried before disinfection or sterilisation, particularly those with narrow-diameter channels. Instruments used on the intact skin surface must be clean.

• *Disinfection* – the destruction or inhibition of pathogenic microorganisms. Endoscopes must be disinfected as a minimum and should be sterile for every procedure. It seems most unreasonable that the first client on a list is examined with a sterile scope while subsequent clients get examined with one that has only been disinfected. In bronchoscopy, for example, sterility is an absolute requirement.

• *Sterilisation* – the complete destruction of pathogenic microorganisms and their spores. Instruments used following surgical incision must be sterile.

Surgery necessitates sterile equipment employed with aseptic technique to minimise the introduction of infection. Most operating departments use sterile services facilities and have on-site provision to 'flash' or 'cold' sterilise items, all of which need regular maintenance to ensure that local standards for sterilisation procedures are maintained.

Sterilisation techniques

Gamma irradiation
Powerful ionising radiation (source Cobalt 60) guarantees sterility and is used on drugs as well as prepacked items of equipment, e.g. sutures, tubing and syringes. Gamma irradiation is very expensive and is managed commercially within secure facilities because of the health risks associated with exposure to radiation.

Steam sterilisation
Although totally inappropriate to modern practice, boiling water is still acknowledged as the cheapest method of sterilisation; the process can be lengthy and damaging to some items. Devices that increase the temperature of the steam make the sterilisation process more efficient by reducing the length of time that instruments have to be 'cooked'.

Water will boil at 100°C but placed in a sealed container from which the steam cannot escape, its temperature rises: the pressure cooker principle. The higher the pressure, the higher the temperature. The autoclave is a sophisticated pressure cooker: steam is retained in a double-walled container, under pressure at high temperatures. On contact with the cold surface of an object, steam condenses; as it condenses heat enters the object. Moist heat kills microorganisms and spores by changing (denaturing) their protein structures. Once the destructive heat cycle is complete a drying cycle is required as retained moisture might become a focus for recolonisation by microorganisms.

Traditional autoclaves work on the principle of downward air displacement. The removal of air allows steam to access all the materials within the autoclave chamber. With valves and door closed, the pressure inside an autoclave rises, associated with which is a rise in temperature. Air is heavier than steam: as valves open to allow steam into the chamber, air is forced down and out of an exhaust port. Once the chamber is full of steam alone and a preset temperature is attained, the exhaust valve closes and the sterilisation process begins. The temperature has to be constant to guarantee sterility. The higher the temperature, the less time required to achieve sterilisation, the minimum being 2 minutes at 32°C, 8 minutes at 125°C or 18 minutes at 118°C at 15–20 psi. These times are significantly increased to ensure that autoclave contents are sterile, as the nature of the loads (even spacing) and choice of packaging can influence even steam penetration.

Once the sterilising cycle is complete, steam has to be removed to prevent wetting of the packs. To stop this cooling and condensation, the autoclave jacket temperature is maintained as the steam is vented; the drying cycle takes 20 minutes. The packs will still be hot when the autoclave is opened and have to be allowed to cool. They then have to be appropriately shelved.

Prevacuum high-temperature autoclaves do not require air displacement as a pump actively removes air from the autoclave chamber; thus the whole cycle is reduced in length.

Autoclaves have inbuilt monitoring and recording devices; their continuous record is vital should any problems arise. Autoclave function is checked with test packs. The 'Bowie Dick' test is used in prevacuum autoclaves; demonstrating an even exposure of the pack contents to steam, it indicates the efficiency of the vacuum pump not the level of sterility. A weekly test with sealed tubes containing spores of a heat-liking bacterium indicates autoclave efficiency. If the bacterium can be cultured from the tube following autoclaving, the autoclave is not working properly and cannot be used until it has been mechanically tested and a 'no growth' spore test result obtained.

Items for autoclaving have to be washed, dried thoroughly and packed. Double wrapping minimises entry of pathogens into sterile packs while on the shelf. Use of an indicator tape or label which demonstrates exposure to high-temperature steam only indicates that the pack has been autoclaved, it does not guarantee the sterility of the pack contents. Labels are used to indicate the exact batch in which instruments were autoclaved, allowing for all instruments in a single batch to be traced.

In theory, items sterilised as described have an indefinite shelf life but many users choose to allocate a shelf life, e.g. 2 years double wrapped in paper, 1 year in linen, etc.

There are occasions when instruments are required quickly and the surgical team cannot wait for a lengthy autoclave cycle (if one were available when needed). There has to be provision for 'flash' or 'cold' sterilisation at close proximity to the operating theatre.

'Flash' (high-speed) sterilisation

These devices operate at around 132°C and 27 psi in the same way as the autoclaves described and are used for unwrapped instruments – they have no drying cycle. The instruments must be thoroughly clean and are placed on a perforated stainless steel tray. Once the steriliser cycle is complete the instruments can be removed using aseptic technique straight to the scrub nurse's instrument trolley. Because the instruments are not wrapped and remain wet, it is imperative that the steriliser is located close to the theatre.

Chemical sterilisation

Used when items cannot be exposed to the great temperatures and pressures generated in autoclaves.

Ethylene oxide (ETO) ETO is particularly useful with moisture sensitive items, for example electronic implants. Sterilisation is dependent upon the gas concentration, temperature and humidity levels and exposure time. Average exposure time is 6 hours but items within an ETO steriliser have to be aerated and that can take 7 days.

There are considerable health risks associated with exposure to ETO; the toxic carcinogen ethylene glycol is formed as ETO combines with water. It is therefore necessary to ensure complete drying of devices sterilised in this way, to protect the recipients of implants and the personnel handling them. The processing of equipment with ETO is also extremely expensive.

Liquid ('cold') methods

Peracetic acid (used with rigid and fibreoptic endoscopes) Fresh peracetic acid has to be used for each sterilising process, making the process very expensive as the recommended immersion time to achieve sterilisation is 10 minutes. Items sterilised in this way require rinsing with large quantities of sterile water before use and must be used immediately.

Formaldehyde Rarely used because it takes up to 24 hours to be effective. It has an unpleasant odour and is believed to be carcinogenic. It is used in low-pressure steam steriliser devices but, by its nature, is damaging and difficult to handle and the sterilisers need frequent maintenance.

Glutaraldehyde Used in a 2% aqueous solution activated by the addition of sodium bicarbonate. Clean items have to be fully immersed for 10 hours in glutaraldehyde before being considered sterile as less than 10 hours will not kill spores. Following immersion, instruments must be thoroughly washed with sterile water before immediate use.

Glutaraldehyde is more commonly used to disinfect equipment; clean equipment must be fully immersed for a minimum 10 minutes to achieve disinfection. Users must abide by strict local policy to ensure that acceptable standards are maintained when using glutaraldehyde.

Users of glutaraldehyde must protect themselves from direct contact with the solution or inhalation of its fumes. Glutaraldehyde must be managed in covered containers with exhaust/extractor devices.

Before using any method of sterilisation, employers should identify and control risks to the health of their employees. For example:

1. provision of heat-resistant protective gloves for use with hot autoclave trolleys;
2. provision of gas masks where there may be accidental emissions from ETO or formaldehyde sterilisers;
3. provision of goggles, masks, nitrile gloves and gowns for use with glutaraldehyde.

The success of these measures is dependent, of course, on employees using what has been provided.

UNIVERSAL PRECAUTIONS

The principles of universal precautions are well established and have been known for many years (Gerberding 1993, Taylor 1993, Cockroft & Elford 1994). However, patients are sometimes still treated on the basis of their infective status (Cockroft & Elford 1994).

Universal precautions work best when they are combined with the principles of risk assessment. Using this system, the level of protection from contamination is based on all the factors involved in the situation. This could include, for example, the risks of contamination when undertaking a particular task, the risks associated with particular infections (such as the incidence of infection and the severity of illness which it causes), the types of task being undertaken, the qualification and experience of the member of staff undertaking the tasks and so on.

The central principles around which this system revolves are as follows.

1. Individuals (in this case all theatre users and patients) must be protected from contamination with all organic matter (such as blood, body fluids, tissues, etc.) (Gershon et al 1994).
2. The level of protection required should be assessed using the principles of risk assessment (Bauer 1991, Telford & Quebbeman 1993, NATN 1998).

Universal precautions policies should cover every aspect of operating department work relevant to infection control: for example, cleaning and maintenance, entrance and exit of personnel, disinfection of equipment, use of protective clothing, use of masks and management of accountable items. The policy should also be integrated closely with any hospital infection control policies and with the various relevant departmental policies.

An implementation plan will ensure that staff are prepared for the introduction of the policy and will smooth the necessary changes which will need to be made. This may include education programmes to update staff regarding the process of risk assessment, the writing of protocols and the rationale behind the policy.

A major factor to take into consideration regarding resourcing of the system is the subjective and generalised nature of some of the behavioural changes (e.g. wearing of masks or gloves) and the lack of access to true costs (because of budgetary inadequacies). A pilot of the policies for a period of time may be useful in order to assess the cost implications on the basis of use of the items (Pobanz 1989) or behavioural changes; for example:

- glove costs – unsterile and sterile;
- surgical face masks;
- costing of a regular maintenance programme;
- breathing circuits;
- a specific number of single-use items, e.g. diathermy blades, suction liners;
- audit of changeover times.

Risk assessment in infection control

The format of the NATN Risk Assessment Guide (NATN 1997) can be used as a basis for the risk assessment process (Fig. 2.1). In the context of universal precautions this can be taken to be assessing the risks associated with contamination, i.e. the possibility of contamination and the severity of the infection if it occurs. The possibility of contamination can be assessed using audit in the clinical setting, for example by auditing the number of needlestick injuries received while undertaking a particular task. The risks associated with infection can be assessed from relevant research, government figures, current opinion, experience and so on. The severity of the infection can be based on the infectivity of the organism and the seriousness of the illness which it produces.

For example, the chance of coming into contact with a patient infected with variant CJD is currently very small (Steelman 1994, Advisory Committee on Dangerous Pathogens 1998); this incidence can be monitored through sources such as DoH figures and of incidence reports. The impact of actually getting the disease is very high, since mortality appears to be around 80% and the causative organism is infective by several routes and is also extremely stable and resistant to many sterilising methods (Steelman 1994). However, the overall risks are very low as there is almost no chance of coming into contact with the disease from a member of the general public. This incidence may rise when considering specific groups such as neurosurgical patients (Advisory Committee on Dangerous Pathogens 1994).

Criterion: The activity to be measured

	Sample	Sample	Sample	1	2	3	4	5	6	7	8	9	10	This is the number of times the activity is measured
Yes			1											= Total. This is number of times an event occurred (i.e. likelihood)
No	0													= Total. This is number of times an event didn't occur
N/A		X												= Total. When it is considered inappropriate to record the event

Impact

Likelihood	Score taken out of number of applicable events from above table
Impact	Assessment of impact if it actually occurs (range = 0–4 (low–high))
Risk score	Score (= likelihood x impact)

Figure 2.1 Risk assessment form.

Therefore, when the patient is not considered to be at risk (i.e. in a high-risk group) of having CJD, there is no point taking the precautions required to protect individuals against infection from this particular organism. If the patient has a suspected or known infection of CJD then the precautions taken should be extreme and could include, for example, burning instruments, destroying theatre equipment, initiating longer sterilisation cycles and so on. This strategy is based on the current understanding of the low incidence of the VCJD prion.

On the other hand, the risks associated with contracting hepatitis B virus (HBV) or human immunodeficiency virus (HIV) are much higher because the incidence in the population is higher (therefore the chance of coming into contact with a patient infected with HBV or HIV is high) and the impact of getting the diseases is also high as they can cause serious illness or death (Montecalvo et al 1995). This means that, from the point of view of HBV or HIV risk, precautions should be taken against contamination by organic matter from all patients regardless of their infective status.

From this, it can be concluded that staff should be protected from contamination with the organic matter of all patients and also that where an infective state is known or suspected, specific advice may need to be obtained from an expert in infection control regarding the protection from infection with that particular organism.

Protocol forms can be used to encourage some standardisation of practice where situations are routine – for example, cleaning of theatres (Fig. 2.2). The use of the protocol forms includes carrying out a risk assessment of the situation, describing the range of protective clothing or the specific actions required and then distributing the protocol around the area for general use.

One of the major benefits which occurs with a major change towards universal precautions is the rethinking of policies and practices which may not have been questioned in years. A major problem with infection control policies is sometimes the tendency to provide strict guidelines which do not allow for a flexible approach to problem solving. Adopting the principles which have been outlined above allows for all the factors to be taken into consideration. A policy based on these principles also encourages individuals to assume full accountability for their practice.

Example 1

Description of situation
Washing contaminated instruments in a sink following an operation

Risks identified
High risks associated with needlestick injury – high probability of it occurring and high impact if it does occur because of the high risk of bloodborne infection
Splashing to face
Contamination of theatre clothing

Protective clothing required
Goggles
Mask
Surgical-quality gloves
Plastic apron

Action required
Sharp instruments/items to be washed individually
Learners not to wash instruments until given proper instruction
Instruments only to be washed by person placing them in sink

Example 2

Description of situation
A major operation for a patient with a known infection of HBV

Risks identified
High probability of major blood spillage affecting gowns, drapes and theatre environment
Possibility of needlestick injury (with high risk of infection with HBV)

Protective clothing required
Scrub staff – standard theatre dress, mask, goggles, double gloves, disposable gown
Circulating staff – standard theatre dress, mask, gloves

Action required
Members of staff should have gone through an immunisation programme
Individual tasks should be assessed for risk of contamination by organic matter and appropriate protective clothing used
Equipment/items in the immediate area should be protected from contamination or removed

(Because of the high incidence of bloodborne viruses such as HBV, the above precautions need to be taken for all major cases, regardless of infective state.)

Example 3

Description of situation
A minor case where the patient is HBV positive

Risks identified
Risk of needlestick injury

Protective clothing required
Standard theatre dress for all staff – additional protective clothing as required

Action required
Assess each task to ensure that the appropriate protective clothing is used each time in order to avoid contamination

(Because of the high incidence of bloodborne viruses such as HBV, the above precautions need to be taken for all minor cases, regardless of infective state.)

Figure 2.2 Examples of protocol forms.

REUSE OF SINGLE-USE ITEMS

Reuse or recycling has received considerable attention since single-use items became commonplace. Baxter (1986) discussed how single-use items had emerged to reduce the toil of perioperative practitioners. She described the complex nature of surgical equipment and how difficult it is to dismantle, disinfect and sterilise. She also noted that swabs were no longer recycled in the UK, because it is impossible to totally eradicate protein debris from their fibres. Baxter (1986) recommended a comparison between the potential costs of 'reprocessing', to save money, and the potential cost of litigation. Ultimately, she identified that the onus lies totally with the practitioner who chooses to recycle an item as a manufacturer has only to indemnify a single-use product for its first, and to their knowledge only, use.

Nothing has changed since 1986, yet still users persist in recycling single-use products. The laws governing all products sold for use in any situation are the Sale of Goods Act (1979) and the Supply of Goods and Services Act (1982) which require items sold to be 'fit for their purpose'.

All goods are required to be used within their manufacturer's instruction. If a user deviates from the instructions they must accept responsibility when things go wrong. This applies equally to someone assembling a device for use in the home and someone preparing an instrument for use during surgery.

Where an item is opened in error or is not used, having been opened, the only recourse is to approach the supplier to arrange repackaging and sterilisation or replacement, but this might involve significant expense.

If single-use items are recycled, primary responsibility lies with the practitioner who packages and sterilises the item or who dictates that reprocessing should take place. If an employer is aware that such practices occur and does nothing to stop them, the employer must accept vicarious liability. If employers can prove that they were unaware of the practice, individual practitioners involved bear total responsibility. Even with the knowledge of an employer's vicarious liability, the individual practitioner must accept personal responsibility and be accountable for their practice.

The legal onus rests entirely upon the individual who decides to recycle an item. Items designated 'single use only' have been so labelled for a reason. The person recycling the device would have to prove that, in reprocessing, the device has not been changed, damaged or altered in any way.

Once an item has been opened and repackaged the manufacturer bears no liability for its subsequent performance. Just consider whether you personally would rather have 'brand new' or 'second-hand' and apply that thinking to the recycling of single-use items. Consider also what a patient, given the choice, would choose.

Back in 1986, Baxter recommended informing patients that funds were insufficient to purchase single-use products, in the hope that patients' rights organisations would lobby to secure adequate funding and put a stop to this poor practice. To date, the problem remains. There is hope on the horizon, in the unfortunate guise of Creutzfeldt–Jakob disease which is known to be caused by a prion, a protein which adheres to tissues – nervous tissue and white blood cells particularly. As Dyke (1997) points out, the prion is known to be resistant to all acknowledged forms of sterilisation. Universal precautions are employed to offer all patients the same standard of care and level of protection, no matter what their infection status. In future, all surgery might be conducted with disposable instruments in an attempt to prevent the spread of the disease. In this event, it would become negligent to recycle instruments.

INADVERTENT HYPOTHERMIA

In some types of surgery (e.g. cardiac) it may be a requirement to lower the body temperature but generally it is more likely that loss of body temperature is unintended and this is known as inadvertent hypothermia. Bernthal (1999) suggests that up to 90% of patients experience hypothermia in some way during the perioperative period.

Hypothermia is classified according to three stages:

- Mild: 33–35.5 °C;
- Moderate: 30–33 °C;
- Severe: below 30 °C (NATN 1998)

Heat loss generally occurs through four main mechanisms:

- Conduction: the transfer of body heat directly to colder objects
- Convection: through moving air currents
- Radiation: the transfer of heat to colder objects nearby
- Evaporation: the heat utilised during conversion of water to vapour

These factors combine with a number of others that might occur during the perioperative period, including the following.

- Long periods of preoperative fasting that inhibit metabolism.
- Immobility.
- The effects of anaesthetic agents, e.g. peripheral vasodilation which transfers heat from the core to the shell of the body. Depressed hypothalamic response to heat loss such as the shivering response. Also, due to unconsciousness the patient loses the ability to respond to heat loss in a behavioural way such as adjusting the room temperature or clothing.
- Ambient theatre temperatures, which are often kept low to suit the comfort of the staff.
- Length and type of surgery.
- Emergency surgery.
- Unnecessary exposure of the patient, e.g. before the surgical team are ready to commence surgery.
- The use of room-temperature intravenous fluids.
- The very old and the very young, or patients undergoing emergency surgery, are at more risk of heat loss during surgery.

The consequences of inadvertent hypothermia may be dramatic. Low body temperature may be responsible for postoperative shivering which can increase oxygen consumption by 100–400% (Kruse 1983, Ciofolo et al 1989); this contributes to arterial hypoxaemia and can have dire consequences for the patient. Shivering also impedes monitoring devices and can cause distress to patients and strain the surgical wound. Slotman et al (1985) found that low body temperature following surgery has been associated with cardiac arrhythmias, respiratory failure, sepsis, wound dehiscence and death.

It has been found that ambient theatre temperature and the age of the patient are the most important indicators of temperature loss during surgery (Hind 1994).

The prevention of inadvertent hypothermia should be the goal of perioperative care and a variety of measures should be employed to achieve this goal.

- High-risk patients need to be identified and appropriate steps taken to specifically reduce the risks to these patients. This will include the young and the old, in particular patients under 10 and over 60 years old, as well as patients undergoing emergency surgery.
- Patients should be kept covered with appropriate clothing and blankets throughout the entire perioperative period. This might include the use of thermal ('space') blankets or 'forced air' warmers where indicated or available.
- Temperature monitoring should be undertaken as a routine observation and this should also be recorded on the patient's perioperative records.
- The use of intravenous fluid warming techniques should be considered when large amounts of room-temperature fluids are being given.
- Ambient theatre temperature should be kept between 21 and 24 °C.

- Operating departments should set standards for minimising the risks of inadvertent hypothermia.

PREVENTION OF PRESSURE SORES

Preventing pressure sore development is an important part of ensuring quality care and patients in the perioperative environment are clearly at risk of pressure sore development.

Bridel (1993) defines a pressure sore as an area of necrosis caused by excessive and prolonged pressure. There are many factors responsible for pressure sore development in perioperative patients.

- Older patients are more at risk due to diminished integrity of the skin and support structures.
- Thin and emaciated patients due to poor protection of bony prominences.
- Obese patients due to poor tissue perfusion and the extra risk of shearing forces whilst being moved.
- Long periods of immobility throughout the perioperative period. In particular, the 'forced immobility' whilst the patient is unconscious.
- Poor nutritional status.
- Dehydration.
- Shearing forces and friction during movement and excessive tilting of the operating table.
- Poor positioning.
- Circulatory and metabolic changes during anaesthesia.
- Inadvertent hypothermia causing cell hypoxia.

Clearly, many of these factors can be identified in individual patients and measures taken to reduce the risk of pressure sore development. These might include:

- identification of high-risk patients through effective assessment processes and the use of a pressure sore risk assessment tool (e.g. Waterlow Scale 1988);
- avoiding lengthy fasting periods preoperatively;
- safe handling and careful positioning of all patients;
- avoiding too much tilt on the operating table;
- the use of pressure-relieving mattress and other aids during surgery;
- implementing a system for monitoring pressure area care throughout the perioperative environment.

INTRODUCTION OF NEW TECHNOLOGY INTO THE OPERATING DEPARTMENT

The future belongs to change: continuous change, development, expansion, invention. And technological change is becoming the greatest factor in shaping work practices (Handy 1993). One of today's popular micro-processors, the pentium chip, is built on a tiny piece of silicon, roughly the size of a fingernail. It weighs about the same as a cube of sugar and uses less than 2 watts of electricity. This chip can execute over a billion instructions every second. Around 50 years ago, one of the first modern computers was capable of executing around 5000 instructions per second and used 140 000 watts of power. This is progress. If the car had progressed as quickly as this, it would be possible to buy one for less than £10 and travel from Edinburgh to London in less than an hour for around 50p (Pritchett 1994).

The phenomenal development of computer power has been equalled by developments in almost every other area. The result is that as soon as a piece of equipment comes out, it is obsolete. Or, at the very least, it has been superseded by yet another piece of equipment with even more bells and whistles.

This has several implications for theatre staff who must:

- constantly learn, unlearn and relearn new skills;
- understand principles as well as specifics;
- be aware of the implications associated with accepting new equipment (Surkitt-Parr 1997).

Learn, unlearn and relearn

At one time, the introduction of a piece of new equipment was a rare event. There would no doubt be a lot of input into its introduction, time to assimilate and investigate what it could and couldn't do and, once in place, many years in which to practise using it. This is no longer the case. New equipment and techniques come out on a daily basis, new techniques appear constantly. What was true yesterday may not be true tomorrow. All this means that people have to be prepared to learn quickly and put that knowledge into practice almost instantly. After a particular length of time, that knowledge and skill will become obsolete, at which point the person then has to unlearn the old skills in order to relearn current skills.

This constant change can be very traumatic and destructive unless managed properly. Negative results will be a fear of new technology and a psychological unplugging which can lead to dangerous or unnecessary practices (Lindsay 1997).

Case study 2.2

I heard an orthopaedic surgeon say to a patient, 'You can have an operation where we look down a tiny telescope and try and see what the problem is or we can open up your knee and do the job properly'. The surgeon was describing an arthroscopic operation to a knee, a procedure which would have been less traumatic for the patient and would have resulted in a shorter stay in hospital. He had never learned how to do this particular operation or use that equipment. (See p. 123 for details of the legal implications.)

Understanding principles

Understanding principles means that the individual is prepared for change. Consider, for example, the original diathermy machines. These early machines were practically identical to the machines produced today, insofar as the surgical effect is concerned. The difference is in their monitoring systems. Modern electrosurgical generators have sophisticated alarm systems which can detect error conditions so that, in effect, accidental burns should be a thing of the past. However, accidental burns still occur. If they are not due to equipment malfunction, which is extremely rare, then they must be due to human error and this is often the case. In so many situations, there are no wrong or right answers or wrong or right ways of doing things. There are just better or worse ways. The two main areas to consider, therefore, are how to use the equipment effectively and efficiently and how to prevent harm to the user or the patient.

Electrosurgery

The use of electrosurgery is a classic example of the advances in technology (Wicker 1992, 1997, 1998). The modern electrosurgical generator is

Table 2.2 Some principles associated with the use of electrosurgery

Principle	Implications for practice
High-frequency electric current is used to heat body tissues	Since heating of tissues is the purpose of the equipment, by definition it must be dangerous to use. Electric current by its nature is difficult to control.
Concentration of the electric current leads to an increased heating effect	The return electrode must have sufficient contact with the patient to prevent concentration of the current. Small active electrodes will cause a more intense heating effect. They are therefore more suitable for cutting than desiccation.
Every electric current requires a circuit in order to flow	If the circuit is broken current will stop flowing. If one circuit is broken, the current will pass along the path of least resistance in order to find another pathway.
High-frequency electric current behaves like radio waves	Radio waves are transmitted through the air therefore electrosurgery current could also be transmitted through the air – this happens when 'open keying' the active electrode.
Capacitance occurs due to the magnetic field around electrodes	Gloves do not need holes in them in order for the wearer to get an electric shock. It is not good practice to coagulate blood vessels by touching the active electrode to a haemostat.
High voltage leads to the formation of sparks	High-voltage waveforms are best for coagulating large areas of bleeding.
Low-voltage waveforms are less likely to produce sparks	Low-voltage waveforms are safer because of the low incidence of sparking. Low-voltage waveforms are better in minimal access surgery where the extent of accidental burning may go unnoticed.

a computer-controlled electrical generator which produces a high-frequency electrical output. There are so many applications where electrosurgery is used, areas of the body where an electrosurgery burn could occur and situations in which it could arise that there is really little point in describing specific ways in which to avoid burns. It is much more effective to teach the principles by which electrosurgery works, so that the user is able to identify areas of concern and then act on the information.

That it has been used for almost a century in surgery does nothing to prevent electrosurgery from being abused and misused by people who are not aware of its potential and limitations. Table 2.2 illustrates the use of principles in guiding good practice and in avoiding harm.

The implications of accepting new technology

Individual nurses are accountable for their own practice. If nurses use a piece of equipment without knowing how it works or how to avoid the dangers of its use, then they will be personally accountable for problems which arise. It makes sense, therefore, to have a protocol for the introduction of new technology (see Box 2.1).

Education

It is essential that an education programme is put into place alongside new technology in order to ensure that the equipment is used safely, to its maximum effect (see Box 2.2).

The manufacturer is often best placed to provide an education programme and this is something which can be negotiated on purchase.

Box 2.1   A protocol for the introduction of new technology

Education
What it does
How it does it
What are its uses
What are its dangers

Policy and procedure
How to set it up and check it
How to clean and maintain it
How to use it safely and efficiently
Remedial actions to take if something goes wrong

Quality assurance
A standard for its use
An audit of its use

Risk assessment
Identification of risks
Precautions required

Manufacturers' handbooks and guidelines are also a very good source of information. As a minimum, any education programme should have information on:

- what it does
- how it does it
- what are its uses
- what are its dangers.

Box 2.2   Outline lecture plan for the use of electrosurgical equipment

---

What is electrosurgery?
- Radiofrequency electrical current
- High frequency

How does it work?
- Mains frequency current is converted into radiofrequency (RF) current
- RF current heats the tissues as it passes through them

The three surgical effects
- Desiccation
- Fulguration
- Cutting

Monopolar electrosurgery
RF current
  - Components of the electrical pathway
Circuit
  - Earthed
  - Isolated

Electrosurgical waveforms
- Coagulate
- Cut
- Blend

Bipolar electrosurgery
- Active and return electrodes part of forceps
- Current path only between tines of forceps
- No patient return electrode

Hazards of electrosurgery
- Thermoelectric burns
- Electrocution
- Interference with electromedical equipment
- Smoke inhalation
- Explosion/ignition

Alternative pathways
- Wet drapes
- Drip stands

- ECG electrodes
- Rectal thermometers
- Steinmann pins
- Mayo stands

Return electrodes
Functions
- Disperse the current
- Safe pathway out of the patient
Principles
- Choose well-vascularised muscular mass
- Avoid bony prominences, skin lesions
Problems
- Peeling off
- Defective
- Not plugged in
- Alternative pathway chosen by current
- Not big enough
Solutions
- REM
- Active electrode monitor

Minimally invasive surgery
Direct coupling
- A nearby instrument becomes active
Insulation failure
- Insulation (out of sight) is defective
Capacitive coupling
- Non-conductor separated by two conductors

Safety checks
- Plugs, sockets and mains lead
- Foot pedals
- Active electrode and lead
- Return electrode and lead
- Patient

Policies and procedures
The function of a policy in this context is simple – to apply a standard to the use of a particular piece of equipment. The procedure will inform individuals about the recommended method of use.

Policies should be written with the help of the manufacturer's information and input from the users. It is essential that both the policy and procedure are seen as being effective and useful in the working situation (see Box 2.3).

Quality assurance
In the context of this section, application of the principles of quality assurance will ensure that a credible standard of use is established and maintained through the application of standard setting (Table 2.3) and auditing (Table 2.4).

Box 2.3   A policy and procedure for the use of electrosurgical equipment

---

The electrosurgical generator (diathermy machine) is responsible for 3% of all medical negligence claims involving hospital staff. In Scotland during the years 1981–91 this amounted to 26 cases of accidental patient burning. This is likely to be the tip of the iceberg as many such burns never get reported.

It is therefore imperative that all theatre staff using this equipment are familiar with its use. The first defence against accidental patient burns is a knowledgeable and skilled staff.

Documentation
All operating departments should have:
- a copy of theatre safeguards;
- a copy of the manufacturer's manual for the generator in use in that theatre;
- information regarding the safe use of electrosurgery. As a minimum this should include:
    - *Working with electrosurgery* (NATN) and/or
    - 3M booklet on electrosurgery and/or
    - ValleyLab's booklet on electrosurgery and/or
    - Journal articles related to electrosurgery and/or
    - Any other relevant information;
- a copy of recent hazard notices relating to the use of electrosurgery.

General maintenance
- Ensure that the generator is part of routine maintenance check by the medical physics department.
- Routinely check all electrical cables and the general condition of the control panel, plug and switches. Report any faults or damage immediately.

Before use
- Ensure that the machine is clean and has no obvious faults or damage.
- Check that the generator is functioning correctly as per the manufacturer's handbook. As a minimum this should include:
    - check the alarm system prior to the patient's arrival in the operating department;
    - ensure that the insulation on the cables is intact;
    - if the plate is reusable, ensure that it is clean and in working order.
Please note: most generators have more than one alarm system (for example, patient voltage monitor; patient plate monitor; patient earthing monitor) so make sure that you know how to test for each alarm. The instructions for testing the alarms are in the manufacturer's manuals.

During use
- Ensure that all connections to the generator are made before switching it on.
- Shave excess hair before applying the plate.
- Make sure that the patient is not touching any earthed metal objects.
- Ensure good contact between the patient and the plate, over an area of good muscle mass.
- Check the plate if the patient is moved during surgery.
- Place the plate as close as possible to the operative site.

Box 2.3 cont.

- Check all connections if a power increase is called for.
- Check the patient for contact with earth if a power increase is called for.
- Keep active electrode clean during use.
- Always use an insulated quiver.
- Never coil the return electrode cable when it is in use.
- Beware of any modification to existing equipment.
- Make yourself familiar with the equipment in use.

After use

- Always check the patient's skin at the site of the return electrode for signs of damage.
- Wipe footpedals with warm water and detergent without immersing them fully in water.
- Keep the active electrode in the quiver until the generator is switched off. Never lie the active electrode on an earthed surface (for example, a metal trolley) while the generator is switched on as this can lead to patient burns.
- Never reuse a single-use return electrode.

Conclusion

Constant vigilance is required in order to avoid accidental patient burns. As a minimum, make sure that you are aware of how the generator works and the safety checks which the manufacturer recommends prior to its use.

Table 2.3 A standard for the use of electrosurgery

Standard statement: The risk of harm to the patient during the use of electrosurgery will be minimised

Structure	Process	Outcome
A policy is available in the operating department regarding the use of electrosurgical equipment	The nurse will be given instruction before using the equipment. The nurse will record all accidents which occur with electrosurgery	The patient will be protected from poor practice during the use of electrosurgery. Patient safety will be monitored
Information is available about the safe use of electrosurgery	The nurse will be able to demonstrate a working knowledge of the equipment	Patient safety will be ensured by the appropriate use of the equipment
An inspection programme is carried out by the medical physics department	The nurse will ensure that all equipment has been properly maintained before its introduction into the operating department	The patient will be protected from faulty equipment
The correct equipment will be clean and available for use when required	The nurse will check all equipment before use	Patient safety will be enhanced by the use of appropriate equipment

Table 2.4 Audit tool on the use of electrosurgical equipment

Criterion	Source of information	Yes	No	N/A
All equipment is clean	Observe (OBS)			
No inflammable anaesthetic gases are in use	OBS			
A team member is designated to check the equipment	OBS			
Manuals are kept for equipment in use in theatre	Document			
Regular maintenance is carried out	Document			
The wall socket is checked for damage before use	OBS			
The plug and lead are checked for damage before use	OBS			
The footpedals are checked for damage before use	OBS			
The scrub nurse checks the insulation on the instruments before use	OBS			
The return electrode is placed on an area free from hair	OBS			
The return electrode is placed on an area free from lesions	OBS			
The return electrode is fastened securely to the patient	OBS			
The return electrode is placed over an area of large muscle mass	OBS			
The return electrode is used as per the manufacturer's instructions	Document/OBS			
The patient is protected from metal contact with earth	OBS			
The return electrode is connected correctly	OBS			
The live electrode is connected correctly	OBS			
The power setting is checked by the surgeon in charge	OBS			
The patient's skin is checked postoperatively	OBS			
Damage to the patient's skin is recorded as per policy	Document/OBS			
Damage to the patient's skin is reported to the hospital administration	Document/OBS			
The ward nurse is informed of any damage to the patient's skin	OBS			
The staff are instructed in the use of diathermy	Ask nurse			
The staff are instructed in the dangers of diathermy before use	Ask nurse			

These principles ensure that the best techniques are used, with the minimum impact on patient and staff care and safety (NATN 1998).

Risk assessment

The principles of risk assessment are detailed in Chapter 6. A risk assessment exercise will identify factors such as staff training, equipment maintenance and untoward incidents which will help to identify a strategy for reducing risks (NATN 1997).

The ever-increasing use of highly technical equipment in the anaesthetic room has made it essential for nurses to be proactive during its introduction into the operating department. The alternative is misuse of equipment with potential dangers for staff and patients.

CONCLUSION

The culture in which nurses work today is very different from that of only a few years ago. Patients now know more, expect more and are prepared to use the law if things go wrong.

Nurses have at their disposal the tools with which they can protect themselves and their patients, through risk assessment and management and the use of evidence-based practice.

Care documentation is vital: when things do go wrong, investigation can take months; it may be years before a case reaches court. Individual use of reflective diaries affords practitioners even more protection as they have a method of recalling 'untoward' events.

The ultimate 'protection' is to be perfect and always to work within the rules. Secondary to that is the need for adequate insurance, a vital resource in perioperative practice where there is so much opportunity for things to go wrong.

REFERENCES

Advisory Committee on Dangerous Pathogens 1994 Precautions for work with human and animal transmissible spongiform encephalopathies. Health and Safety Commission, London

Advisory Committee on Dangerous Pathogens 1998 Transmissible spongiform encephalopathy. Health and Safety Commission, London

Barker A, Cassar S, Gabbett J 1994 Handling people: equipment advice and information. Disabled Living Foundation, London

Bauer P 1991 Universal precautions in our practice. Part 1: of risks and regulations. Nursing Management 22(8): 56Q–56X

Baxter B 1986 To reuse . . . or not to reuse, that is the question. NAT News February: 18

Bernthal E 1999 Inadvertent hypothermia prevention: the anaesthetic nurse's role. British Journal of Nursing 8(1): 17–25

Bridel J 1993 Pressure sore risk in operating theatres. Nursing Standard 7(32): 4–10

Ciofolo M, Clergue F, Devilliers C, Ben-Ammar M, Viars P 1989 Changes in ventilation, oxygen uptake and carbon dioxide output during recovery from isoflurane anaesthesia. Anaesthesiology 70: 737–741

Classification, Packaging and Labelling Regulations 1984. HMSO, London

Cockroft A, Elford J 1994 Clinical practice and the perceived importance of identifying high risk patients. Journal of Hospital Infection 28(2): 127–136

Consumer Protection Act 1987. HMSO, London

Control of Substances Hazardous to Health Regulations 1988. HMSO, London

COSHH revision occupational exposure limits 1994. HMSO, London

Daily Mail 1998 The crazy world of compensation: doctor's $\frac{1}{2}$ million pounds for trauma of pricking her finger. October, 10

Dimond B 1995 Legal aspects of nursing, 2nd edn. Prentice Hall, London, ch 2, p 29–36

Display Screen Equipment Regulations 1992. HMSO, London

Domin M A 1995 Hepatitis C: sleeping giant among bloodborne pathogens. Personal communication

Dyke M 1997 Creutzfeldt–Jakob disease – an emerging risk. British Journal of Theatre Nursing 7(8): 33–35

Environment Protection Act 1990. HMSO, London

Gerberding J P 1993 Procedure-specific infection control for preventing intraoperative blood exposures. American Journal of Infection Control 21(6): 351–356

Gershon R R M, Karkashian C, Selknar S 1994 Universal precautions: an update. Heart and Lung: Journal of Critical Care 23(4): 352–358

Handy C 1993 The age of unreason. Business Books Ltd, London

Health and Safety Executive 1991 The manual handling of loads: proposals for regulations and guidance. HMSO, London

Health and Safety at Work Act 1974. HMSO, London

Hind M 1994 An investigation into factors that affect oesophageal temperature during abdominal surgery. Journal of Advanced Nursing 19: 457–464

Hutt G 1994 Glutaraldehyde revisited. British Journal of Theatre Nursing 3(10): 10–11

Kruse D 1983 Postoperative hypothermia. Focus on Critical Care 10(2): 48–50

Lindsay L 1997 Just tell me . . . which knob do I press to cancel the alarm? British Journal of Theatre Nursing 7(5): 21

Management of Health and Safety at Work Regulations 1992. HMSO, London

Manual Handling Operations Regulations 1992. HMSO, London

McFarlane I 1995 Whose back is it? British Journal of Theatre Nursing 4(11): 8–12

Montecalvo M A, Sung Lee M, DePalma H, Shein Wynn P E, Lowenfels A B et al 1995 Seroprevalence of human immunodeficiency virus 1, hepatitis B virus, and hepatitis C virus in patients having major surgery. Infection Control and Hospital Epidemiology 16(11): 627–632

National Back Pain Association and Royal College of Nursing 1997 Guide to the handling of patients. Introducing a safer handling policy. National Back Pain Association, Middlesex

NATN 1997 Risk assessment guide. National Association of Theatre Nurses, Harrogate

NATN 1998 Principles of safe practice in the perioperative environment. National Association of Theatre Nurses, Harrogate

NHS and Community Care Act 1990. HMSO, London

Occupational Exposure Standards 1994. HMSO, London

Personal Protective Equipment at Work Regulations 1992. HMSO, London

Pobanz R 1989 The economic impact of universal precautions on a surgical unit. Nursing Management 20(1): 38–42

Pritchett P 1994 New work habits for a radically changing world. Pritchett & Associates, Dallas

Provision and Use of Work Equipment Regulation 1992. HMSO, London

Sale of Goods Act 1979. HMSO, London

Seymour J 1995 Counting the cost. Nursing Times 9(22): 24–27

Slotman G, Jed E, Burchard K 1985 Adverse effects of hypothermia in postoperative patients. American Journal of Surgery 149: 495–501

Snell J 1995 Raising awareness. Nursing Times 9(31): 20–21

Steelman V 1994 Creutzfeldt–Jakob disease: recommendations for infection control. American Journal of Infection Control 22(5): 312–318

Supply of Goods and Services Act 1982. HMSO, London

Surkitt-Parr M 1997 The role of the nurse in the adoption and diffusion of new technology. British Journal of Theatre Nursing 7(9): 33–35

Taylor M 1993 Universal precautions in the operating department. British Journal of Theatre Nursing 2(10): 4–7

Telford G, Quebbeman E 1993 Assessing the risk of blood exposure in the operating room. American Journal of Infection Control 21(6): 351–356

UKCC 1989 Exercising accountability. United Kingdom Central Council, London

UKCC 1992 Code of professional conduct. United Kingdom Central Council, London

Waste management: the duty of care code of Practice 1991 HMSO, London

Waterlow J 1988 Calculating the risk. Nursing Times 83(39): 38–60

Wicker P 1992 Making sense of electrosurgery. Nursing Times 88(45): 31–33

Wicker P 1997 Electrosurgery. In: Shephard M, Mason J (eds) Practical endoscopy. Chapman & Hall Medical, London

Wicker P 1998 Principles, uses and hazards of electrosurgery. In: Clarke P, Jones J (eds) Bridgen's operating department practice. Churchill Livingstone, Edinburgh
Workplace Health, Safety and Welfare Regulations 1992. HMSO, London

FURTHER READING

Babb J R 1994 Methods of cleaning and disinfection. British Journal of Theatre Nursing 3(10): 12–14

Branson M 1995 Hazards of sharps disposal. British Journal of Nursing 4(4): 193–195

Burns J 1991 Safety first: the key consideration. Professional Nurse 7(3): 183–187

Butrej T 1996 You only get one back! Managing manual handling risks. The Lamp 52(11): 12–15

Clarke P, Jones J (eds) 1998 Brigden's operating department practice. Churchill Livingstone, Edinburgh

Dixon R, Lloyd B, Coleman S 1996 Defining and implementing a 'no lifting' standard. Nursing Standard 10(44): 33–36

Domin M 1998 Highly virulent pathogens: a post-antibiotic era. British Journal of Theatre Nursing 8(2): 14–18

Dyke M 1996 Why not wear gloves? British Journal of Theatre Nursing 6(6): 14–17

East J 1992 Implementing the COSHH regulations. Nursing Standard 6(26): 33–35

Fullbrook S 1998 Legal aspects of the re-use of single use items. British Journal of Theatre Nursing 8(3): 37–39

Green R 1996 Positioning the patient for surgery. British Journal of Theatre Nursing 6(5): 35–38

Jagger J, Bentley M B 1997 Injuries from vascular access devices: high risk and preventable. Journal of Intravenous Nursing 20(65): 533–537

McCluskey F 1996 Does wearing a facemask reduce bacterial wound infection? A literature review. British Journal of Theatre Nursing 6(5): 18–20, 29

Menzies D 1995 Glutaraldehyde – controlling the risk to health. British Journal of Theatre Nursing 4(11): 13–15

Plowes D 1995 Reusing or mis-using? British Journal of Theatre Nursing 5(1): 22–23

Roger D, Nash P 1995 A threat to health. Nursing Times 91(22): 27–28

Shelmerdine L 1995 Occupational asthma: assessing the risk. Nursing Standard 10(4): 25–28

Thomlinson D 1991 Everything starts with a risk rate. Cleaning, disinfection and sharps disposal sterilisation techniques. Professional Nurse 6(7): 386–390

Willmer S, Willson P D, McGuteagark K, Rogers J 1997 Reuse of single use items in minimal access surgery. British Journal of Theatre Nursing 7(3): 11–13

Education for practice

Jane H Reid

Over the decades, dynamism, innovation and change have been intrinsic features of health services and nowhere more so than within perioperative care environments. In the White Paper *The new NHS: modern, dependable* (DoH 1997), the government made clear its commitment to rebuilding public confidence in health provision, emphasising that future health policy will be concerned with promoting interprofessional collaboration, efficiency, effectiveness, excellence, quality, responsibility and accountability across services.

The common denominator to these key concepts and arguably the means to achieving them is education. But most importantly, education and learning must be viewed and accepted by practitioners as a lifelong commitment for no single episode of education will ever be an absolute or sufficiently transferable to every clinical situation.

In the 1980s it was predicted that 'lifelong learning' would emerge as a new phenomenon because it would prove too difficult for people to survive in a society that faced change as rapidly as ours without learning new things.

> When life was simpler, one generation could pass along to the next generation what it needed to know, to get along in the world; tomorrow was simply a repeat of yesterday. Now the world changes faster than the generations and individuals must live in different worlds during their lifetimes . . . (Cross 1981, p. 1)

Given that the unique and vulnerable needs of the surgical patient may be described as one of the few 'constants' in a perioperative care setting, this chapter provides practitioners with an overview of the central features to facilitate education for and in practice.

SUPPORTING LEARNERS IN THE PERIOPERATIVE ENVIRONMENT

The range of personnel that engage in the delivery of perioperative care is considerable, incorporating a multiplicity of skills, qualities and competencies, with each person playing a crucial role in the provision of safe efficient care.

When assessing how learning and skills acquisition might be facilitated in the perioperative environment, it is perhaps important to initially consider the traditional or commonly held images of those who engage in study.

With the historical emphasis on preparatory education programmes for health care, the terms 'student' or 'trainee' invariably conjure up impressions of persons engaged in foundational education, to achieve the necessary competence to practice. In parallel with the concept of 'lifelong learning' and in recognition that practice changes constantly, it is more appropriate to adopt the broader term 'learner'. As a descriptor, 'learner' conveys a universal image, of someone who is in pursuit of knowledge or seeking command of a new skill, regardless of age or position within a hierarchical organisation. The term can therefore be seen as equally applicable to the novice student nurse seeking insight on the preoperative checklist, as to the most experienced perioperative nurse seeking proficiency in a newly marketed joint prosthesis and the associated instrumentation.

Regardless of a person's role and their individual contribution to care within the perioperative cycle, all should be considered as having learning needs at varying points along their career. Recognising that learning is a universal need makes it easier to create the right environment to make it possible.

Creating a learning environment
Why?

In examining why it is necessary to create and maintain a learning environment in the workplace, it is important to understand the legal responsibilities owed to patients and staff by both the employer and individual employees.

All care workers have a responsibility in law to ensure that they are competent, knowledgeable and safe in respect of the specific care afforded to patients. Staff are also required to provide such care with regard to the safety of the environment and the safety of others (see Chapter 2). Nurses, in addition, are professionally accountable for maintaining and developing their knowledge and expertise and further assume accountability for the actions of those to whom they have delegated care (UKCC 1992a,b). Equally importantly, employing authorities are vicariously liable for the standards of care and competence of employees.

The relationship between education, evidence-based care and quality is well recognised, as is the relationship between employer and employee in the provision of appropriate client care. Awareness of these relationships highlights the continuing debate about the purpose of learning in health care.

- Is education designed to safeguard and protect the client from negligent care?
- Is education designed to safeguard and protect the organisation from risk and liability?
- Is education concerned with the pursuit of knowledge, professional autonomy, personal development, fulfilment and achievement of the individual?

Perhaps it is about a synergy of all three and the route to creating a learning environment in a clinical setting is to recognise the relationship and interdependence of each with the other.

Patients, organisations and the professions need education in order to respond and adapt to the relentless pace of change, in terms of advancing technology, health-care demands and the potential of perioperative care provision.

The aim of a learning environment can be defined as maximising all possible opportunities that enable and encourage individuals to master the activities and skills that are fundamental to their sphere of practice, in a manner that:

- gives regard to the rights of individual patients and colleagues to be safeguarded from harm;
- supports the rights of the organisation to be protected from risk;
- supports the rights of the learner to determine the pace and extent of their learning;
- adapts to the demands of contemporary care delivery.

How?

It has long been acknowledged that clinical environments have an atmosphere that can help or hinder learning (Orton 1981, Jacka & Lewin 1987). The challenge in a perioperative care setting is for staff to be aware of the factors that hamper and discourage learning and to optimise that which specifically encourages an individual to progress.

To achieve a good learning environment, emphasis should be placed on negotiation and securing a balance between the needs of learners as well as the needs of the service (the worst feeling in the world is to feel like just a pair of hands!).

The benefits of teamwork and open communication have been highlighted as providing learners with the opportunity to discuss and examine clinical issues arising from practice, emphasising the links between theory and what is actually being experienced (Kenworthy & Nicklin 1989). The contribution that confident qualified staff can make when identified as 'facilitators' to specific learners has been consistently demonstrated as fundamental to providing a learning environment (Morton-Cooper & Palmer 1993).

Optimum learning may be further encouraged by highlighting the many learning opportunities in a given area. Attention should also be given to the individual teaching and learning styles of both facilitator and learner in order to further encourage a supportive environment and facilitate effective working partnerships.

Another important consideration is to acknowledge that learning occurs in a social context. Learning is therefore very dependent upon the values, attitudes, opinions, group norms and group processes of a care team. The positive or negative experiences of the learner as they work with others are likely to have considerable influence upon the way in which they learn and, overall, their perception of perioperative care delivery (Lovell 1990).

Valuing the learner for what they can individually contribute to the care process will do much to boost their self-esteem and confidence in mastering the learning task. The pressures for efficiency of service and optimum patient throughput, often against a perennial backdrop of staffing shortages, are well known. The challenge to the perioperative team in creating a learning environment will undoubtedly involve assessing and balancing the demands and needs of the learner with the continuing demands of service provision.

The opportunities for structured learning away from the immediate clinical setting are rare luxuries in contemporary health care. Perioperative teams are therefore encouraged to recognise the scope of 'teachable moments' (Brookfield 1987) and develop a commitment to a learning culture within the workplace where all occasions in which colleagues could learn from one another are identified.

Too often, teaching and learning are framed in a formal context, with the subsequent risk that staff view themselves as 'too busy to teach'; this results in the educational richness of the perioperative setting being overlooked. It is vital that staff recognise that learning can occur through a variety of interpersonal transactions (see Box 3.1) which should be used to their optimum advantage (Jarvis 1983).

Box 3.1　Learning through interpersonal transactions (adapted from Jarvis 1983)

- Through self-direction
- Through facilitation
- By being taught
- By being instructed
- By being trained
- Through discussion
- Through critical reflection (recall and analysis)
- Through living
- Through role modelling
- By being socialised
- By being influenced
- By being conditioned
- By being empowered
- By being indoctrinated
- By being challenged
- By being supported
- By adapting to circumstances
- Through observation

Meeting learning needs

Whilst there are universal needs of all learners, such as respect and support as mentioned earlier, and individual learning needs such as pace and preferred learning style, it is also necessary to make distinctions between the purpose of learning and the desired learning outcomes for discrete learner groups.

Meeting the needs of persons engaged in preregistration studies

The appropriateness of preregistration learners gaining experience in the operating department has been one of the most long-standing debates within nurse education and was further fuelled with the introduction of Project 2000.

The majority of preregistration learners continue to be encouraged to gain insights into perioperative care via ad hoc patient 'follow-throughs' from surgical placements. There is evidence that more lengthy placements in either day surgery or the operating department are also being encouraged by educationalists, so providing learners with the opportunity to gain greater experience in previously 'undervalued' areas of practice.

NHS reform and policy in the late 1990s demanded that a primary care-led NHS should prevail. Whilst such developments are already evident, the first decade of the 21st century will continue to witness a major shift in health-care resourcing and a fundamental change in the balance between hospital and community care. Surgical intervention and perioperative nursing care will continue to be key features of acute care delivery, with a polarising of services between new-style high-technology centres and community-focused provision. However, it is vital that the elements and tradition of perioperative care are celebrated and made explicit for preregistration learners.

In anticipation of further technological and anaesthetic advance and the continuing development of ambulatory surgery, there is increasing scope for more care in GP procedure rooms and day care centres. From the standpoint that education is about ensuring that people are 'fit for purpose', the challenge for perioperative staff is to educate preregistration learners about the fundamental aspects of perioperative nursing care, regardless of the environment.

The goal for preregistration learners is to gain competence in nursing skills and to develop insights into and understanding of the tradition of caring. Whilst we cannot predict the future of nursing or indeed where nursing will be carried out, nurses will continue to:

- coordinate care;
- teach carers, patients and professionals;
- maintain a special concern for the ill and vulnerable as well as those who are currently well;
- provide technical expertise and skill.

The diversity and richness of perioperative practice provides the opportunity for preregistration learners to gain valuable experience. It is up to care teams to value the perioperative tradition, advertise it and establish healthy alliances with educational institutions which will affect placement opportunities.

Meeting the needs of persons engaged in postregistration studies

The key demand for nursing in contemporary health care is adaptability. The extent to which an individual nurse can adapt in order to address changing practice demands is dependent upon the manner and the pace at which nurses can develop and enhance their knowledge and skills. Change generates a cycle that perpetuates the need for practitioners to be committed to 'lifelong learning'.

It is important to distinguish between the types of study nurses may engage in when considering postregistration studies. First, the UKCC (1992a) mandates that all professional nurses re-register periodically and that they provide a minimum portfolio of evidence which demonstrates that they have engaged in learning to maintain their competence in specific aspects of professional practice.

There will also be a rotation of staff new to perioperative care who will be required to gain proficiency in perioperative procedures and clinical skills. Technological advances will continue to present their own educational challenges. There will also be some who, having taken career breaks, find themselves described as nurse returnees, eager to refresh once-honed skills. There will also be a proportion of the nursing team who wish to accelerate their careers and recognise that a possible route to this is advanced study.

In order to foster a learning culture in the workplace, all postregistration study must be recognised as equal. Both management and clinical staff should be discouraged from valuing certain courses or units of study over others, as this can lead to tension between staff and, in particular, anxiety or embarrassment for those who may be seeking support (funding or study time) for their specific learning needs.

All learning should be recognised as credible and uniquely valuable to the individual member of staff concerned, for it builds upon their existing skill and knowledge and enhances their contribution to the delivery of perioperative care.

PROFESSIONAL DEVELOPMENT PROGRAMMES AND LEARNING NEEDS ANALYSIS

Conducting a learning needs analysis (LNA) is arguably the key to planning any individual's further study. The value of LNAs and their relevance to all staff cannot be overestimated. They are more commonly associated with continuing professional education as opposed to preregistration study, because the curricula in preregistration education are driven by achievement of specific outcomes at certain points of a programme associated with competence to practice. On registration, however, specific factors challenge the qualified nurse and these include:

- the diversity and dimensions of perioperative practice;
- the need to maintain professional competence;
- the need to master new skills;
- the need to expand the scope of traditional practice spheres/adopt new roles;
- professional accountability;
- the pace and stress of the workplace;
- a need to balance domestic and professional demands.

Perhaps more importantly, there is a need to recognise that all persons learn at different rates and will have different priorities. There is a risk that without a LNA, an individual will feel like a floundering ship on the high seas, struggling valiantly to chart a safe course with no clear idea whether they are headed in the right direction.

LNAs, quite simply, are concerned with identifying learning needs pertinent to the role and grade of an individual staff member and identifying 'key result areas' which require professional development/training for an individual member of staff. On the basis of such information, LNAs assist in the devising or mapping of a personal development programme that seeks to optimise the educational opportunities available in, or in association with, a given environment to assist the staff member to achieve their 'key result areas'.

LNAs can be initiated formally through an individual performance review (IPR), in consultation with a line manager, or they may be devised through discussion with an identified education/training officer within a unit. Similarly and less formally, individual nurses may become aware of their specific learning needs and personal goals through critical reflection, action planning and maintenance of a personal profile.

Above all, personal development programmes should be unique, tailored to an individual's learning needs and incorporating a full range of recognised learning strategies: self-directed study, formally approved programmes of study and work-based learning.

The goal for the individual is to chart a purposeful programme of learning that aids personal development and facilitates enhanced clinical practice.

Where LNAs are generated through critical reflection and action planning, it is important that adequate personal records (i.e. the personal portfolio) are maintained, outlining the scope of the development programme and its relationship to specific 'key result areas'. Rigorous documentation of how learning has developed an individual, contributing to new insight or new skill, may be submitted as evidence of personal updating for PREP.

CAREER MAPPING

LNAs and professional development plans lead on to the concept of career mapping as they provide opportunities to critically assess personal performance and determine a developmental route for an individual to pursue.

It has long been recognised that nurses are not proactive in planning their careers and fail to recognise that they can enjoy significant control over their future, if they take responsibility in planning their development. Traditional ideas of careers as something planned, carved in stone, continuous and lifelong are outdated. Contemporary practice demands that nurses are committed to their development, resourceful in their working methods, flexible and self-reliant.

Career mapping (no more than a 5-year plan at any one time) should be viewed as essential by those nurses who wish to avoid the threat of redundancy. A review of the past decade alone emphasises the extent and significance of change, in particular in terms of how, where and by whom care is delivered. The forecast (DoH 1997) is that the drive for change will accelerate. It is important that perioperative practitioners recognise the limits of vertical career progression but keep an eye on the future and engineer their own careers, which may demand a lateral move into the community.

SUPPORT ROLES TO FACILITATE LEARNING

Whilst the fundamental concepts of perioperative nursing (empathy, hope, pain, empowerment, spirituality, therapeutic touch, presencing, holism, reassurance, caring) are universal and unchanging, the technical aspects of perioperative care have become increasingly complex. Advancing technology, health reform and the rapid throughput of patients combine to create a challenging working environment for even the most experienced of nursing staff.

In environments of challenge, change and demand, it is vital to maximise the scope of human potential by empowering people and optimising their motivation, via supportive frameworks that meet the needs of both the individual and the employing organisation. Supportive frameworks, both formal and informal, have been shown to enhance motivation, encourage creativity, stimulate risk taking, nurture developing leadership qualities and benefit patient care (Morton-Cooper & Palmer 1993).

Helping relationships generated through a range of support roles can be classified as providing learning, general or emotional support which can assist nurses in practice in a variety of ways (Box 3.2).

Box 3.2   Types of support

Learning support assists nurses to:
- identify learning needs;
- take personal responsibility for meeting learning needs;
- map out a career path;
- appraise personal performance and assess its contribution to achieving organisational aims;
- discover themselves;
- make sense of experiential learning;
- critically reflect in and on practice.

General support assists nurses to:
- communicate effectively;
- reduce absenteeism;
- bolster morale;
- avoid burnout;
- feel good about their work;
- build professional relationships in the workplace.

Emotional support assists nurses to:
- deal with the stress and distress of nursing practice;
- cope with the anxiety and turmoil of change;
- recognise and understand triggers of emotion.

A clear strategy should exist in the workplace that makes it explicit to all staff that support frameworks operate on a principle of reciprocity. The perioperative team should be encouraged to recognise how support can be provided or accessed dependent upon the demands and needs of individuals at a given time.

A support framework (Fig. 3.1) needs to be sufficiently diverse and flexible to take account of the many transition periods and developmental needs that may arise throughout an individual nurse's career (including specific support of preregistration learners, the newly qualified and those experiencing role change).

A range of support roles are common to perioperative practice and utilised to facilitate clinical learning.

Mentorship

Originating from the Greek classics and Homer's *Odyssey*, the concept of mentorship is commonly recognised as a partnership between an inexperienced individual and a more senior, well-respected, expert colleague of the same practice world.

The use of mentorship, predominantly in preregistration nursing, has not been without its critics. It is frequently described as a misused label referring to a predesignated qualified member of staff, charged with the responsibility of supervising a specific learner during a given clinical

Career status   **Nature of learning support and development offered**

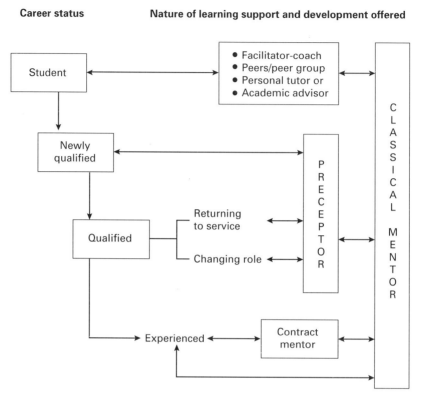

Figure 3.1 Support framework.

placement. It is likely that in the true sense of mentorship, nurses will have few mentors throughout the course of their careers as, once established, the relationships stand the test of time, placement rotations and career moves.

Clinical assessors

The term 'clinical assessor' has evolved as a preferred term in more recent years, better describing the supportive but assessment-focused relationship commonly experienced in clinical practice. As with mentorship, clinical assessors are typically more experienced colleagues who seek to provide learners (both pre- and postregistration) with a broad range of helper functions. However, the title further acknowledges the role played in assessing a learner's performance against predetermined criteria and learning outcomes.

Preceptorship

In 1993 the UKCC issued a position statement that all newly registered nurses, midwives and health visitors and those returning to practice after a break of 5 years or more should be provided with a period of support of approximately 4 months by an experienced practitioner.

The demands and role change associated with the transition from student to professional practitioner have long been recognised, as has the evidence that support and guidance from the more experienced can affect the ease with which individuals are able to assume the responsibility of primary practice. The terms 'preceptee' (newly registered nurse or returnee) and 'preceptor' (experienced nurse) are used to describe those who enter into this supportive relationship.

With regard to professional accountability, the UKCC (1993) made it explicit that the preceptorship period should not be viewed as an extension to the formal programme of learning that prepares individuals to register and that the preceptee will always be considered accountable for their actions, on registration. The UKCC advise that local management should give due consideration to the level of responsibility expected of individuals and recommend that this should be balanced with the experience of the individual.

Recognising the complexities of the perioperative environment, there is much to be gained in ensuring that preceptorship programmes are implemented and that the potential for inappropriate demands to be made of the less experienced is avoided. The provision of support and guidance to facilitate role transition, education of nurse returnees or even the rotation of team members through the disciplines of perioperative care can encourage confidence, enhance self-esteem, contribute to improved motivation, minimise unnecessary stress in the workplace and facilitate due care and protection of patients.

Coach

Another role to appear in recent years to complement the mentorship and clinical assessment function of a supportive framework is that of the coach.

Nursing is about the acquisition and development of caring skills and interpersonal exchange. Linked to the sporting world, coaching is associated with the provision of support and instruction and through individual monitoring, positive feedback and continuous appraisal of practice, the learners' skills are developed.

Coaching, suggests Kelly (1992), is also commonly associated with team effort. The idea that the learning needs of individuals are met to allow them to contribute to an improved team effort accords well with the team culture of the perioperative environment.

Facilitator

In relation to clinical supervision and reflective practice, the support role of the facilitator has also become widely recognised. The experiential technique of 'reflecting on action' provides scope for facilitators to utilise a range of interpersonal techniques (attending, listening, mirroring, paraphrasing and reflecting back) to encourage further analysis on the part of an individual supervisee. Skilled facilitation has the potential to lead a supervisee to new insight and new learning in a safe supportive relationship.

Strategies to facilitate learning

When examining how we can facilitate learning in the perioperative environment, it is appropriate to consider the many different types of knowledge that have to be assimilated by perioperative practitioners to affect safe competent care.

1. 'Know how' knowledge, e.g.:
   - how the diathermy machine works;
   - how muscle relaxants work.
2. 'Know why' knowledge, e.g.:
   - why patients are fasted preoperatively;
   - why information giving promotes patient compliance with health advice and empowered choice.
3. 'Know that' knowledge, e.g.:
   - surgeon X prefers McIndoe scissors for dissection;
   - specimens require double bagging before transport to the laboratory.

All elements of perioperative practice can be thought of in these three ways and the most appropriate strategy to aid the acquisition of such knowledge can then be identified.

PERIOPERATIVE RESOURCES

The greatest resource within the perioperative setting is the team itself. The range of expertise and depth of knowledge commanded by colleagues should be recognised, highlighted and celebrated. Staff with a particular interest in a given area should be encouraged to take a lead role for their subject, educating and sharing their skill and knowledge with others. It is important that the requirements of clause 14 (UKCC 1992b) are appreciated by all staff and that responsibility for the education of colleagues is viewed as implicit in the professional role.

In recognising that people are the richest teaching resource in a clinical setting, it is equally useful to remember that people can have a detrimental effect upon the learning process. The power of role modelling cannot be overestimated and all staff have a responsibility to ensure that they practise ethically, safely and within the parameters of protocols and agreed standards at all times.

Teaching and learning demand resources other than people and the relationship of education with practice and efficient, effective care demands appropriate funding.

It is recommended that staff have access to facilities to aid their development. These should include:

- books, journals and literature pertinent to the practice discipline available within the immediate environment of the department;
- quiet room (that could contain a library resource of staff projects and assignments undertaken by staff);
- access to a library/study centre;
- access to IT facilities for on-line searching, use of the Internet, computer-assisted learning;
- visual aids to facilitate teaching: video, OHP (overhead projector), white board, flip chart, slide projector and screen.

SELF-DIRECTED LEARNING

It is necessary to remember that learning can be achieved without formal teaching and specific instruction. Self-directed learning arises from an individual's natural curiosity and questioning approach or from individuals being made aware (reflection on and in practice) of a deficit in their knowledge and skills.

It is presumed by educationalists that learners engaged in formal units of study (particularly postregistration) take responsibility for their learning and make themselves aware of the associated study aims, objectives, learning outcomes and assignment requirements. Such structure provides sufficient guidance and direction to enable learners to focus their attention and enquiry along a particular path of study.

A noteworthy situation related to preregistration learners or those new to perioperative practice concerns the possibility that persons 'may not know what they don't know'. This does not mean that people cannot take personal responsibility for the pace and focus of their learning but that they will often benefit from advice and guidance regarding the priorities and sequence of their study programme.

Appraising practice

In recent years there has been an increasing emphasis on examining practice through self/peer analysis and discussion. Reflective techniques such as reflective practice and critical incident analysis enable practitioners to recognise and understand:

- how and why things may have happened in a particular way;
- the need to explore what emotions and values influence the way in which people behave in a given context;
- the relationship of theory to practice.

The goal of reflection is that learning and care enhancement result from an appraisal of clinical decision making and personal performance and that through the process of analysis, new insight is reached to inform future practice.

The stress and demanding nature of perioperative practice, in particular 'out of the ordinary' events (an intraoperative death or major incident), further demand reflection and analysis. Following situations where the outcome was unexpected or not favourable, staff are often left feeling upset and uncomfortable, wondering if their personal contribution or the team effort could have effected a more positive outcome.

Debriefing is a useful strategy to assist staff to explore the reason for their stress and anxiety and to understand the reason for their emotions. Unresolved stress and burnout are recognised causes of attrition across the nursing service. Whilst the goal of debriefing is to provide emotional and psychological support, the analytical process can also prove a valuable learning strategy, contributing to an individual's emotional growth and the identification of coping and self-management strategies that may be put to good effect on future occasions.

Journal clubs

It is often suggested that nurses are poor readers. With increasing emphasis on evidence-based care, perioperative teams may wish to consider the benefits to be gained by establishing a journal club in the workplace.

Monthly meetings over lunch periods, during which staff take rotational responsibility for reporting and sharing material from the wider literature, should be encouraged as a useful and informative learning strategy. The range of material that can be reported is vast, including local research, DoH circulars, UKCC position statements, material accessed from the Internet and the professional journals, to list but a few.

Recognising the pressures of the perioperative environment, a journal club can contribute effectively to the updating and informing of many through a shared but minimal effort.

CONCLUSION

Education for practice is an essential element of professional development, synonymous with the concepts of quality, standards of care and professional accountability. With the growing emphasis on clinical effectiveness and evidence-based care, the dynamism of the perioperative environment demands that practitioners continually appraise and reflect on the currency of their knowledge base. As such, there needs to be an emphasis on *current learning* and/or *future learning*, compared with a dependence on *past learning*, for the trends and techniques of today need to be recognised as the likely rituals and traditions of tomorrow.

REFERENCES

Brookfield S D 1987 Developing critical thinkers – challenging adults to explore new ways of thinking and acting. Open University Press, Milton Keynes
Cross K P 1981 Adults as learners. Jossey Bass, San Francisco
Department of Health 1997 The new NHS: modern, dependable. HMSO, London
Jacka K L, Lewin D 1987 The clinical learning of student nurses. King's College, University of London
Jarvis P 1983 Professional education. Croom Helm, London

Kelly K J (ed) 1992 Nursing staff development: current competence and future focus. Lippincott, Philadelphia

Kenworthy N, Nicklin P 1989 Teaching and assessing in nursing practice. An experiential approach. Scutari Press, London

Lovell B 1990 Adult learning. New patterns of learning. Routledge, London

Morton-Cooper A, Palmer A 1993 Mentoring and preceptorship. A guide for support roles in clinical practice. Blackwell Science, Oxford

Orton H D 1981 Ward learning climate. A study of the role of the ward sister in relation to student nurse learning. Royal College of Nursing, London

UKCC 1992a The code of professional conduct, 3rd edn. United Kingdom Central Council, London

UKCC 1992b The scope of professional practice. United Kingdom Central Council, London

UKCC 1993 Registrar's letter. The Council's position concerning a period of support and preceptorship: implementation of the post-registration education and practice project proposals. United Kingdom Central Council, London

FURTHER READING

Dean D 1996 Leadership and you. Nurses need to plan their careers to take on leadership roles. Nursing Management 3(1): 8

Morton-Cooper A, Palmer A 1993 Mentoring and preceptorship. A guide for support roles in clinical practice. Blackwell Science, Oxford

Perioperative communication

Maureen Dyke

INTRODUCTION

Communication is the exchange or sharing of information between two or more parties. Although it can take many forms, the concept remains the same. Communication is central to human life but is often taken for granted and may suffer in quality as a result.

High-quality perioperative communications are essential to support the main aims of perioperative nursing, including the delivery of high-quality patient care, ensuring the safety of staff, efficient management of the department and ensuring ongoing professional practice and development. In relation to patient care, it is particularly important because of the relatively short time available to interact with patients, especially when they are likely to be apprehensive.

TYPES OF COMMUNICATION

Written

Examples of written communication include documents, policies and protocols, operating lists, off-duty rotas, induction programmes, educational material, courses/study days and professional organisation notices. The list is, of course, almost endless.

The presentation of the written word is important because words are powerful tools and can be easily misinterpreted, with catastrophic results. Several factors should be considered since communication is a two-way process and it is not only the delivery but also the reception which is important. Written communications should be welcoming, not threatening; eye catching, not dull; informative and easily understood, not written in academic or management jargon.

Verbal

This is the area that many people think of when considering communications. The actual language used, its tone, relevance and timing are of equal value. When information is exchanged and the speaker is angry, timid or frustrated, there can be an adverse impact on the listener. Timing is particularly applicable during surgery. For example, information may go unheard or only be half remembered if the receiver of the information is talking to a patient or is in the middle of an intricate procedure.

Listening is the equally important other half of any verbal communication. Listening involves concentrating on what the speaker is saying, looking interested and not interrupting. This is a skill that requires practice as it is so easy to only half listen. This is partly due to the fact that the spoken message is relayed at a slower rate than our ability to listen, thus allowing time to concentrate on something else (Reece & Brandt 1987). Asking questions to clarify the message should not be automatically regarded by the speaker as a sign that the other party is not listening or does not understand. Instead, it should be seen as a sign of the level of interest, responsibility and respect for the message giver.

Developing a good telephone manner is imperative to efficient verbal communication. This applies to both parties. The speaker needs to adopt good clear diction to ensure the message is understood, particularly as body language cannot be observed. It is perfectly acceptable for the receiver of the message to ask for it to be repeated or to repeat it back.

Another form of verbal communication is the 'grapevine'. It is widely recognised that the information gained from this source is not always accurate and can lead to misunderstanding, but research has revealed that it is accurate 75% of the time (Aldag 1985, cited by Strader & Decker 1995). It does provide information that may not be available from official sources and often at a faster rate. According to Boyd (1995), it can be strong in impact and subtle in the way it works. Gossip might also be included under this heading. Perioperative nurses are no different from many other groups in society and where the gossip remains non-malicious, it is fairly harmless.

Non-verbal

Communications may need to be non-verbal as low noise levels are often required, particularly when anaesthesia is being induced or intricate surgery being performed. There is therefore a need for non-verbal communications in perioperative practice.

Sign language during surgery has developed to a highly sophisticated level and is usually acquired by practice and example. Many operations can be conducted with the minimum of speech, particularly when they are without complications. A hand held out will receive the correct instrument, swab or suture. A similar arrangement between the scrub team and the circulating staff also exists. For example, items held up will indicate that further supplies are required or need to be removed from the sterile field. Each team will have its own variation of non-verbal language.

Body language, particularly the use of facial expressions, plays a major part in non-verbal communication. Seeing a friendly, welcoming face (with mask removed) helps patients to cope with their fears. The way we position our bodies says much to indicate how we feel towards one another. Particular stances may indicate a friendly open nature, boredom, dislike or fear. Facial expressions are frequently used in the perioperative setting, despite the use of surgical masks which tend to obscure the face. Raising of eyebrows, smiles, frowns and shaking of heads are all part of everyday language but take on particular significance where speech is discouraged.

Communicating by touch can complement or even replace speech. Many patients will appreciate a hand being held whilst awaiting the start of general anaesthesia or during a procedure using local or regional anaesthesia. It is necessary to develop judgement to recognise when this is not welcome. A comforting hug for a colleague who has had good or bad news or just a difficult day or a friendly handshake to a new member of staff all play their part in developing good tactile communication.

Appearance could also be considered since this area is difficult for perioperative practitioners because of the rather shapeless theatre clothing usually provided. That said, it is essential to ensure clothes are clean when meeting patients. The provision of reasonably good-quality theatre clothes in order to present a professional image should be a priority for budget holders.

AREAS OF USE

Practitioner/patient

Communication with patients is an essential part of nursing practice which is learned during training. The development of a good relationship is difficult because the time a patient spends in the operating department is very brief. Preoperative visiting helps to strengthen the rapport between patients and nurses but only if the practitioner also greets and remains with the patient throughout the perioperative period. (Ward visiting does have other benefits and should be encouraged.) An information booklet specifically for patients coming for surgery, preferably written by the theatre staff, is an excellent way of providing better communications, particularly where preoperative visiting does not regularly occur.

Patients should be greeted by name and receiving members of staff should introduce themselves. Documentation is dealt with elsewhere in this book (see p. 125) but when involving patients directly, it should be handled in an efficient and sympathetic way. Many patients come to theatre without their dentures and are too embarrassed to talk. They will often speak with a hand held in front of their mouth, making conversation difficult. The routine removal of dentures before anaesthesia is no longer necessary and should be replaced by a more individualised assessment of need. There can also be problems caused by the absence of reading spectacles or hearing aids, though it is now rare for the latter not to accompany the patient.

Talking down to patients on low beds or trolleys is another bar to good communication and should be avoided by sitting patients up where appropriate or raising the level of bed or trolley. Any strategy to diminish this situation should be used as patients already feel vulnerable.

Patients should never be left alone in the operating suite, either in the reception area or in anaesthetic rooms. An informed member of staff should remain with the patient and attempt to openly answer all questions that are raised. Reassurance is important at this stage as well as the recognition and acceptance of many aspects of behaviour displayed due to fear and apprehension. Some patients do not wish to talk and this should be respected. Trying to establish conversation may be inappropriate after heavy sedation, although even under these circumstances procedures should not start without an explanation.

Where local or regional anaesthesia is used, it is customary for a perioperative practitioner to remain with the patient, holding a hand if this is acceptable or just sitting beside the patient, providing support and company. An explanation should be given that pain during surgery is not to be expected and that the patient should indicate if any discomfort is felt. It is a measure of the practitioner's skill to judge whether the patient wishes to be told what is happening, wants to talk of non-medical matters or not talk at all.

During the postoperative period communications should be established at the earliest opportunity following general anaesthesia. Hearing is usually the first sense to return and an apparently sleeping patient may be aware of conversation. As in the preoperative period, explanations of what has occurred and what is currently happening should be given alongside continuous reassurance.

Practitioner/practitioner

The frequent use of non-verbal communication has been outlined above but this is only one form of the daily interaction between colleagues. Sharing of information about patient care, operating schedules, equipment requirements, both new and in current use, and the support of new members of staff should all be part of day-to-day practice. Mutual support, reassurance and encouragement are as important to our fellow practitioners as they are to patients. Problems should be discussed and solutions sought.

The handover between staff from one shift to the next necessitates good communication. The details required are complex and may include the surgery which is still in progress, operations booked, which team is on call, how many patients are in the recovery area, number of staff on duty and personal crises which may affect practice. More essential is the shared information on the continuation of individualised patient care which should be part of normal daily practice.

Practitioner/manager

This is an area where the two-way process continues to be important. Obviously, the leadership style of the directorate will have a profound effect. Whether democracy or autocracy rules will vary from one department or hospital to another. The provision of unit meetings, where all are allowed their say without interruption or derision, is the ideal. Sharing of information and suggestions for improvement can be discussed in a friendly way. Communications will tend to be one way when a top-down style of management is in practice. However, a well-argued case is more likely to be considered when words are chosen carefully and presented in a non-confrontational way, with appropriate body language. The dissemination of information outside meetings is essential. Minutes should be taken and then made available for those unable to attend and as a reinforcement of what was said for those who were present.

A well-planned education system needs to be implemented when a new and unfamiliar piece of equipment is purchased, as it is totally inadequate to explain it to individuals in the theatre team and expect them to pass it on to everyone else. This often results in staff using equipment in a potentially dangerous manner.

The formation of policies, protocols and procedures is often seen as a management function, unless staff are suitably empowered. There should always be consultation on these matters and it is a failure of the communication process if they are implemented without opportunity for discussion. Different styles of leadership will influence the handling of these issues. Discussion with staff will be the norm when a transformational style is in place whereas transactional leadership has a different style. The work of Bass (1990) provides an insight into the contrasts between these styles.

Policies should be accessible, although this can sometimes be a difficult task. Notice boards are notorious for being overcrowded, out of date, untidy and subsequently unread. Smart folders kept in the manager's office will also remain unread. Each department should have a discussion on communications, the availability of documents and important pieces of information and try to select a method that will result in good dissemination of information.

Practitioner/medical staff

Communications between practitioners and medical staff have had a history of being rather one way, according to Porter (1991). He found that this situation has improved with nurses having progressed 'from their original subservience, through informal covert decision making, to the present time when informal decision making is accepted as a valid nursing strategy'. There is more recognition of teamwork, which has resulted in improved efficiency of operating departments. Discussion of the holistic care of patients throughout their perioperative journey should occur on a regular basis.

Level of nurse seniority and established working relationships can positively affect this interaction. The appropriate timing of communication is essential during surgery and is not a difficult skill to cultivate. It has long been the custom for messages for surgeons to be passed via the scrub nurse. This is a sensible precaution as that person is better positioned to choose the appropriate moment. This is part of the protocol of 'who may speak to whom'. Whilst sounding somewhat old-fashioned, where used sensibly, it ensures good communication between the two disciplines.

Practitioner/others

As in any other hospital department, there is constant communication with other areas, haematology, other laboratories, X-ray, occupational health, infection control, hospital secretaries and the wards. Much of this exchange is via the telephone and the usual rules should apply. It is easy to allow an urgent situation to interfere with good diction, but its absence will only delay a response. A notepad and forms for transcribing laboratory results should always be kept beside the telephone.

IMPROVING COMMUNICATION

Improving communication is part and parcel of the ongoing process and cannot be separated; many factors involved in improving communication have therefore been dealt with as part of the discussion so far. Clear, concise use of language is a priority. This does not mean using short statements or abbreviated language but a careful choice of words, expressed succinctly. Naturally articulate people have few problems in this area, but all can improve with wide reading. Mann (1980) provides excellent guidelines on this subject.

Other factors which should be considered are those related to culture, which may dictate the style of verbal communications. Space between speakers may contribute to the emphasis of the message but also may be governed by culture. Eye contact is another area considered important by some and insulting by others. Other body language may include messages that may be misinterpreted if cultural diversities are not taken into account. The work of Mancini (1995) is worthwhile reading as an excellent short reference to this subject.

Barriers to communication

The use of poor speech has already been discussed as a barrier. Jargon is another common problem and whilst this is inevitable, it is wise to be wary of inappropriate use. It is not usually comprehensible to patients (and new staff), who may be too frightened or embarrassed to admit they do not understand. If the jargon user remembers that not all those with whom they are communicating will understand, then the transmission of 'mixed messages' may be avoided (Mackenzie 1998). Plain English is recommended, but this will not always suffice where there are language difficulties. Each hospital will have local arrangements for translators to be available. A system devised by Gilsenan (1992) suggests how to address this problem in the postoperative area.

Abbreviations come into a somewhat similar category. Again, patients or staff do not always understand them. They should be avoided where possible and should not appear on operating lists or theatre registers. It is probably unreasonable to expect their abolition, though efforts have been made in recent years to decrease their use, particularly on prescription scripts.

Position in the theatre directorate hierarchy can have a negative effect on communication. Those at the lower end of the scale may find it difficult to communicate, particularly if they have reason to be critical of an incident. There should be established lines of communication to assist junior members with this obstacle.

Lack of communication

Lack of communication with patients can lead to their experiencing a higher level of apprehension than necessary. It seems somewhat obvious to state that they should be kept informed, at a level suitable to their understanding. Areas of interest will include anaesthesia, surgery and recovery and how their pain will be controlled.

The level of frustration staff feel when communications are poor can have an adverse effect on their practice. Staff need to feel valued and where this does not occur, morale tends to be low and motivation may decrease.

Assertiveness

The days of nurses having to behave in a submissive, subordinate manner should no longer exist. Research by Sweet & Morton (1995) found that the use of assertiveness by nurses, in the interests of their patients, was fairly widespread and probably due to the improved status of women as well as changes in nurse education. A level of assertiveness is required in order for nurses to practise their role and if this is not part of their character then it can be learned. Most hospital trusts provide suitable courses.

Assertiveness may be a necessary trait for perioperative nurses because of sustained periods of work alongside medical practitioners. For centuries doctors have practised their profession by prescribing care, while nurses supported them and the patients. This medical model still has its supporters but is no longer valid with the move to graduate nurse training, nurse practitioners and nurse-led units. There has been some progress towards the acceptance that all team members play an equally vital role in the delivery of high-quality care. Where this has not yet led to an equitable working relationship, assertiveness may need to be exercised. Timing again needs to be considered when attempting to be assertive.

There may also be problems with senior members of staff. For those who are shy or timid, it is difficult to be assertive when communicating with their manager. They may find discussion difficult, particularly if they wish to comment on some aspect of practice which they find to be detrimental to high-quality care. On these occasions it is sensible to plan what needs to be said, keeping notes of the points to be included and delivering a well-argued case.

The danger of assertiveness is that it may become aggressiveness and there is a fine line between the two. Being assertive means defending personal rights and opinions, whilst aggressiveness includes hostility and may also be offensive. It is very easy, having learnt to be assertive, to slip over into a more aggressive style and alienate colleagues. An excellent comparison of non-assertive, assertive and aggressive communication is illustrated in Strader & Decker (1995, p. 443).

There are a number of books published on this subject and those who need advice can help themselves by studying this aspect of human behaviour, as well as enrolling for a suitable course.

Conflict, challenge and confrontation

Conflict can occur when two or more parties have very different views of a situation. Conflict may develop between parties of similar status or it may be vertical. It can be caused by many factors, including poor communication, work- or home-related stress, difficult working relationships, unsatisfactory staffing levels or change introduced without consultation. In addition, it can be caused by members of staff who persist in being lazy, difficult or obstructive.

Conflict is always bad if it is left unresolved. However, resolved and constructive conflict, resulting in open and frank discussion, may be good as it can influence progress. There is no progress without change and the strategies associated with conflict resolution may be needed to initiate changes that are advantageous in the long term (Marelli 1993, cited by Mackenzie 1998). Changes in patient care, surgical techniques, educational issues related to professional practice and working schedules are some of the aspects where there is continuous progress.

Some practitioners will challenge any new decision. This may be done for a variety of reasons, according to Strader & Decker (1995). These include the personal pleasure that some people derive from being awkward or alternatively it may be done to ensure there is a full explanation and discussion of the proposed change.

The term 'confrontation' is often used in a similar way, although there is frequently a degree of hostility included.

Managing conflict should be done as part of a three-part process of assessment, identification and intervention. In a theatre managers' forum on managing conflict, reported by Wicker (1998), the importance of having a 'no blame' culture was emphasised as being essential for a disciplinary process to be received positively. In any situation it was suggested that it is necessary to analyse the problem by pinpointing the type of conflict and the personnel involved. Issues need to be identified and confined, particularly with regard to priority (Wicker 1998). Anger needs to be managed before the appropriate conflict resolution can be employed.

There are five main styles of managing conflict, according to Swansberg (1993). **Competition** results in a win/lose situation. This may be used where a manager has the power to assert authority and believes this to be the appropriate solution. It will probably not provide a good example of conflict management to the losing party. **Compromise** occurs when one of the two sides relinquishes part or all of their goals. It may be used as a permanent measure if peace can be restored or as a temporary measure until collaboration can be organised. **Collaboration** is achieved when both parties can be reasonably satisfied. It is the ideal solution but requires time, patience and cooperation of those involved. **Avoidance** is the moving away from a situation, usually where anger is present, to avoid further damage. Again, it can only be considered as a temporary measure, which will need resolution when the anger has been diffused. **Accommodation** will work where there is a climate of tolerance between the people involved, who are prepared to discuss their differences amicably and settle on a solution without the need for time-consuming collaboration, but it has limited use.

Bullying and intimidation

This subject is getting much more publicity, though this does not necessarily mean there has been an increase in incidence but rather that it is being recognised and reported as an unwelcome aspect of working relationships. It can take many forms and come from a variety of sources. It is not acceptable for any member of staff to be subjected to this behaviour from another member of staff. Rudeness, a raised voice, belittlement, derision, undermining and threats are all forms of bullying. This conduct can be exhibited by peers, both junior and senior staff, and by doctors. For many years nurses, particularly junior nurses, have accepted this treatment as part of their normal working pattern. It has caused stress, affected performance and self-confidence and has resulted in some sufferers leaving the profession (Graveson 1998).

How this issue is dealt with depends on its extent, source and the qualities of the recipient. Isolated incidents can often be attributed to the stress of the moment and, depending on the circumstances, may be ignored. Where the bullying or intimidation has occurred before and is from a peer, it should be discussed with the manager, who should use conflict resolution methods. Where it is persistent, further measures may be necessary and disciplinary procedures instituted.

Intimidation from senior staff and managers is a difficult situation for a junior member to confront. If the recipient finds it impossible to discuss it with the person involved, steps should be taken to report it as high up the management structure as is required. Guidance from a professional organisation should be sought and if necessary, a grievance process initiated. Excellent advice on this issue is given by Graveson (1998), including national helplines.

The doctor/nurse bullying situation is one with which many perioperative nurses are familiar. This is partly due to the historical nature of their relationship, when doctors ruled and nurses obeyed. Although less common in today's professional practice, it still occurs. Where the behaviour is occurring with junior doctors, it is fairly easily remedied by making clear that this behaviour will not be tolerated. At consultant level it is still not acceptable. It may be possible to tackle the issue by discussion between the two parties, using conflict resolution measures. If there is no improvement, referring the offending party to the appropriate clinical director may be a last resort. Removing the intimidated party from this environment may be deemed sufficient, where the behaviour is perceived as just a personality clash, but even this should be discussed with the people involved to ascertain if there is simple remedial action that can be taken.

A form of bullying in reverse, where the perioperative practitioner does the bullying, was highlighted by Wicker (1998). Examples of scrub nurses hiding favoured instruments from surgeons were given.

CONCLUSION

This chapter has addressed many of the issues related to communication in perioperative practice. It is not intended as a comprehensive analysis of all the many facets of this essential aspect of theatre practice, which would require a volume of its own. It is intended as a springboard to foster an interest in a frequently ignored aspect of professional life. There is a wealth of literature available and both new and experienced perioperative personnel can gain from further reading on this subject.

REFERENCES

Aldag R J 1985 Management. South Western, Cincinatti
Bass B M 1990 From transactional to transformational leadership: learning to share the vision. Organizational Dynamics 18(3): 19–31
Boyd M A 1995 Communications with patients' families, health care providers and diverse cultures. In: Strader M, Decker D (eds) Role transition to patient management. Appleton & Lange, Norwalk, Connecticut
Gilsenan I 1992 Intercultural communication system. British Journal of Theatre Nursing 2(7): 15–16
Graveson G 1998 Workplace bullying: the abuse of power. British Journal of Theatre Nursing 7(11): 21–23
Mackenzie J 1998 Ward management in practice. Churchill Livingstone, Edinburgh
Mancini M E 1995 Managing cultural diversity. In: Vestral K (ed) Nursing management: concepts and issues, 2nd edn. Lippincott, Philadelphia
Mann H E 1980 The nurses' communication handbook. Aspen Systems, Germanton, Maryland
Porter S 1991 A participant study of power relationships between doctors and nurses in a general hospital. Journal of Advanced Nursing 16(6): 728–735
Reece B L, Brandt R 1987 Effective human relations in organizations. Houghton Mifflin, Boston
Strader M K, Decker P J 1995 Role transition to patient care management. Appleton & Lange, Norwalk, Connecticut

Swansberg R C 1993 Introductory management and leadership for clinical nurses. Jones & Bartlett, Boston

Sweet S J, Morton I J 1995 The doctor/nurse relationship: a selective literature review. Journal of Advanced Nursing 22(1): 165–170

Wicker P 1998 Managing conflict: National Association of Theatre Nurses managers' forum. NatNewsletter 90: 3

Quality and quality assurance

Andrea Star

INTRODUCTION

As we move forward in the new millennium, there are many challenges involved in the delivery of health care. In the operating department environment, one of the most important challenges is to make sure that the quality of care is consistently high. Every perioperative nurse should always strive to maintain and improve the quality of care because every decision and action taken will affect someone: a patient, colleague, surgeon, anaesthetist or other staff in departments or wards.

WHY QUALITY?

Quality is fundamentally important to all organisations, whether they are providing services or making and selling products. Delivering quality means that customers become satisfied with the levels of service that an organisation provides. Failure to provide a quality service will, ultimately, endanger the future prospects of an organisation.

Delivering quality care has always been an aspect of health care but it was not until the early 1970s that attention focused on the real importance of quality in a theatre environment. Since then, the concept of ensuring quality of care has gained momentum. Early practice focused on assessing quality through retrospective audits. Today, the emphasis is more on building quality into each task, through processes that encourage continuous quality improvement.

With the inception of Trust status, quality monitoring became a focus for Trust Boards. Various approaches were adopted by different Trusts: some collected data related to specific high-level quality indicators such as patient waiting times, whilst others developed quality strategies that encouraged all areas within the organisation to put in place local quality monitoring arrangements.

Many perioperative nurses who participated in a quality monitoring process used their professional association, the National Association of Theatre Nurses (NATN), to support them in this venture. In 1987 the NATN published its Quality Assurance Tool, a pioneer in the field, and a team of external assessors was put together to assist with its use. In 1994, this document was redesigned to focus the audit trail on the patient's experiences; thus it follows a patient's journey through the operating department. This tool was renamed the Quality Assurance Document, now commonly referred to as QuAD, and is described in more detail later in this chapter (NATN 1994).

The drive for quality in health care has been supported by successive recent governments and is emphasised in the three recent government White papers: *The new NHS: modern, dependable* (England) (DoH 1997a), *Designed to care: renewing the NHS in Scotland* (DoH 1997b) and *Putting patients first: the future of the NHS in Wales* (DoH 1997c). All three White Papers make it clear that future health policy must be designed around a patient-centred health service with a commitment to clinical effectiveness to ensure that patients receive the highest quality of care possible.

Clearly, quality and clinical effectiveness are closely linked concepts. In some senses, the drive for clinical effectiveness is the drive for quality from a clinical perspective.

CLINICAL EFFECTIVENESS

Clinical effectiveness is a term that has recently become fashionable in health care. For many years, quality issues within the operating department have been addressed by a multifaceted approach. Any process to improve the quality of care in theatres will have looked at combinations of the following: audit, research, risk management, complaints monitoring, performance management and education and training. All these factors are now being brought together under the banner of clinical effectiveness.

In 1996 the NHS Executive defined clinical effectiveness as:

The extent to which clinical interventions, when deployed for a particular patient or population, do what they are intended to do, that is, to maintain and improve health and secure the greatest possible health gain from the available resources.

The RCN (1996) subsequently developed an operational definition in which clinical effectiveness is described as: 'applying the best available knowledge, derived from research, clinical expertise and patient preferences, to achieving optimum processes and outcomes of care for patients'.

It is important to remember that clinical effectiveness is essentially concerned with two fundamental issues. Better quality must be translated into both improved patient care and best value for money.

Clinical effectiveness is now being applied to many tasks in health care. The emphasis is on building quality into each and every process. To help in achieving continuous quality, the following principles should be followed. Any process or task should:

- be patient focused;
- be clinically led;
- be multiprofessional;
- ensure access to and sharing of good-quality clinical information;
- be supported by education and training.

Patient focus

This will be particularly important in the care planning process. The named nurse will take responsibility for planning nursing care based on an assessment of individual patient needs. Unfortunately, some theatre nurses view their day's work as a list of surgical cases and forget to think about the individual requirements of each patient undergoing the surgery. In order to avoid this and ensure a patient-focused approach, preoperative visiting enables theatre nurses to undertake the assessment of need and then relate that back to their colleagues so that the individual patient's care can be planned and implemented accordingly (see Case study 5.1). Visits can also be undertaken by theatre nurses in the postoperative period to directly ask patients how they felt about their experience of going to the operating theatre. This will enable theatre nurses to hear about their practice through their patients and make changes where appropriate.

Case study 5.1

Mr Smith was scheduled to have major orthopaedic surgery. He had been admitted the afternoon prior to the date for his surgery and that evening a member of the operating theatre team had visited him as part of the planned preop visiting programme.

Following introductions, the nurse explained to Mr Smith the sequence of events that would occur the next morning as he went through the operating department. This included a description of the anaesthetic room, operating theatre and recovery area and the roles of the different team members, some of whom Mr Smith would meet. After checking that Mr Smith had received a visit from the anaesthetist, the nurse asked him if there were any questions he would like to ask, noting that he seemed very uneasy.

At this point Mr Smith said that his father-in-law had just died and that he was still very upset. He had not mentioned it to anyone because if his operation was cancelled he did not want another long wait on the waiting list. The nurse asked Mr Smith whether he wanted to proceed with his operation and he said he would prefer not to. With this information the nurse was able to inform the surgeon and anaesthetist and a decision was taken to cancel his operation and reschedule it for the following week. Mr Smith was very relieved and satisfied with the outcome.

Clinical lead

Nurses provide patient care throughout the perioperative period. Preoperatively both in patient visiting and in the anaesthetic room; interoperatively in the roles of scrub and circulating nurse; and postoperatively in the recovery room and during follow-up visits. From their education, training and experience, they are able to make informed decisions as to the priorities and appropriateness of this care and support medical decision making through informative communication. By working with others to recount this knowledge, they can make a valuable contribution to the development of a quality strategy.

Multiprofessional

It is accepted that any process auditing the patient's experience of a service needs a multidisciplinary approach including all professional staff who contribute to the patient's treatment and care. This must include nurses, doctors, operating department practitioners (ODP) and operating department assistants (ODA). Teamwork is vital in an operating department and part of that relates to the ability to share knowledge.

Access to and sharing of good-quality clinical information

The monitoring of trends, patterns, improvements and poor performance within an operating department is an essential component which produces reliable and valid information. This information can then form the basis of a strategy to develop a quality monitoring framework which sets targets to demonstrate improvements. Information of this nature can be shared by theatre users to inform practice, shared with managerial colleagues to highlight achievements and shared with perioperative colleagues in other hospitals to compare and identify best practice. 'Benchmarking' is the term commonly used to describe the process of comparing available data against defined performance indicators with other similar-sized hospitals. It can be a useful way of quantifying a department's performance and identifies variants from the average in the benchmarking group. This shows where an operating department is over- or underperforming and in what specific areas of practice. Investigations into these variants both internally and externally (that is, hospital identified as having best results) could lead to changes and improvements in a department's performance.

An example of this process might be an investigation into the rate of cancelled sessions. An operating department with a high rate (commonly greater than 15% of planned operating time) would no doubt wish to examine this further. Common reasons for cancellations are poor communication of annual leave, staff absence and unavailable equipment. Understanding the factors associated with high cancellation levels allows an action plan to be developed to ensure that these factors are rectified, leading to an increase in theatre utilisation.

Education and training

In order for a quality service to be provided, perioperative nurses need to have a full range of skills which are developed through various training and education programmes. In the specific field of quality assurance, training is required for a range of skills for the many processes that enable a practitioner to access, analyse and utilise data to demonstrate the quality of care delivered. Following on from this, additional skills are needed to enable perioperative nurses to set priorities and plan a course of action to solve or minimise the areas identified as poor practice or make improvements to practice.

One development that encourages quality and includes many of these principles is the movement towards more evidence-based care. White

Box 5.1 Four steps to evidence-based practice
1. Formulate a clear question from a clinical problem.
2. Search the evidence for relevant material.
3. Critically appraise the evidence.
4. Implement the findings in practice.

(1997) has shown that this not only improves the quality of the care but also minimises clinical risk factors. Learning from experience and 'trial and error' approaches to care development sometimes wastes valuable resources but also, more importantly, can expose patients to poor-quality care and potential harm. McClarey & Duff (1997) and Smith (1997) suggest that some practices that have not been subject to systematic research persist when their effectiveness is questionable. At present, estimates suggest that only 20% of nursing care is evidence based. The drive for quality and clinical effectiveness means that it is becoming more important to make evidence-based decisions about services. This will ensure that standards of clinical care reflect best practice.

Evidence-based practice is now becoming an important part of the quality agenda in perioperative nursing. Lessons of best practice can be learned and replicated in different situations, always allowing flexibility for particular situations. Four steps have been identified by Long & Harrison (1996) as an approach to evidence-based practice (Box 5.1).

Using the steps outlined in Box 5.1, nurses can systematically examine their activities in caring for patients in order to make sure that they are providing good-quality, cost-effective care.

PATIENT INVOLVEMENT

Recent NHS reforms have placed much more emphasis on involving the patient in health care decisions. The rationale for this is to give patients a greater understanding to help them to make informed choices about their own care. The recent government White Papers explicitly encourage patient involvement in the planning and delivery of their care. This applies in all parts of the health care system, but nowhere is it more vital than in the operating department where nurses undertake an advocacy-type role on behalf of their patients.

Because of this advocacy role, nurses must make sure that they communicate with their patients. Communications skills are contained in all preregistration nursing courses but need constant updating. The greater the opportunities to practise these skills, for example in pre- or postoperative visiting, the more advanced these skills become and the less daunting each episode is. Good communication skills must become part of normal practice.

More specifically, nurses need to collect the views of their patients in order to get an indication of whether patients were satisfied with the care

Table 5.1 Methods of information collection

Source of information	Reason for collection
Preoperative patient visiting	• To plan individual patient care • To meet patient in order to alleviate anxiety • To explain procedures and various staff roles
Postoperative patient questionnaires	• To receive immediate feedback from individual patients about their experience • To evaluate and review practice
Patient focus groups	• To receive considered feedback from individual patients about their experience (usually undertaken by expert facilitators at least a month following surgery) • To highlight common issues arising from the experiences of a group of patients and to produce a shortlist of the main priority areas for action

delivered. This information can be gathered in many different ways. Table 5.1 provides a range of methods.

Each method can provide valuable information from a patient's perspective about their experiences of passing through the operating department. As the nurse trying to measure the quality of care, you need to choose the most appropriate method to get the information you require. You need to bear in mind several factors before involving patients.

• You must ensure that patients are willing to participate.
• You must ensure confidentiality and, where appropriate, anonymity and communicate this to reassure the patient.
• You must be aware of the patient's condition and take this into account when deciding which method to choose.
• You must give a full explanation of the purpose behind and the processes involved in the survey work.

Using any questioning method requires skill and knowledge, not only of the technique but what to do with the data once they are collected. These need to be collated, analysed, interpreted and reported. It is helpful to work with other colleagues and inform your theatre charge nurse who will often be able to offer guidance. It is also important to inform the ward manager as they can provide support and encourage the patients to participate. Report findings should be disseminated as widely as possible, so that others can learn from this work. Useful forums for sharing can include team meetings, seminars and poster displays.

One of the features of the NATN QuAD is that it contains a brief, ready-made questionnaire for patients to complete postoperatively. This can be used as it stands or can be adapted with different questions to meet local need. Figure 5.1 contains the QuAD patient questionnaire.

Patient's number

Please complete this questionnaire and return it to the ward staff. Y (C) means that you agree completely, Y (I) means that you agree but not entirely.

Question	Yes C	Yes I	No	N/A	Comments
Did you receive a visit from a member of the operating department team prior toyour operation?					
Did you feel that the staff prepared you for your visit to the operating department?					
Were you given the opportunity to ask questions?					
Were your questions answered satisfactorily?					
Did all staff introduce themselves to you?					
Did all staff explain what they were about to do to you?					
Did you feel that any pain you experienced was kept at a level which was acceptable to you?					
Were you given an explanation about your care at all stages?					
Was the noise level within the operating department acceptable to you?					
Was the lighting within the operating department acceptable to you?					
Did you feel that your dignity was maintained at all times?					
Total					

Calculation: $\dfrac{\text{Total Yes}}{\text{Total applicable}} \times \dfrac{100}{1} = [\text{SCORE}]$

Figure 5.1 Patient questionnaire.

PROFESSIONAL DEVELOPMENT

Encouraging clinical effectiveness and making sure that patients' needs are met are two vital aspects of delivering quality care. However, they will not be enough in themselves. Equally important is to ensure that the people who provide the care are trained and experienced to the appropriate level. Reference has already been made earlier in this chapter to some of the skills required to develop evidence-based practice.

Quality health care is delivered by professionals who have been educated in both theory and practice. Appropriate skills are learned, practised, mastered and reinforced until they become an integral part of everyday working.

Today perioperative practitioners are qualified via two different routes. Nurses undertake a preregistration diploma course and qualify as registered nurses. ODPs undertake vocational training in operating department practice at NVQ/SVQ level three. Once qualified, a range of courses are available and this is discussed in more detail in Chapter 3.

Because of the changes in requirements for post registration education and practice (PREP) and issues specifically relating to perioperative practice, for example minimal access surgery, continued professional development is essential. This need not only involve designated courses; wider opportunities to learn are available elsewhere. These include attendance at study days, participating in research and audit projects and preparing teaching material for junior staff. In addition, the NATN holds an annual conference with a varied range of educational programmes delivered by perioperative experts for perioperative practitioners. Undertaking any of these activities can contribute to your portfolio of evidence for PREP to enable you to maintain your registration. The conference also affords perioperative practitioners the opportunity to network with other colleagues from across the country to share good practice, resolve difficulties and meet new colleagues.

AUDIT TOOLS AND TECHNIQUES

Quality is a difficult concept to define. A dictionary definition offers; 'degree or standard of excellence, especially a high standard'. In a health service context, quality can be defined as 'a service which gives patients what they need, as well as what they want, and does so at the lowest cost' (Ovretveit 1996).

Some aspects of quality care can be easily defined and measured. Specific standards can be set and criteria identified and a measurement made indicating compliance. Critics would argue that this may mean achievement of a minimum standard with no incentive to improve (Williams 1994).

Other aspects of quality are difficult to assess: for example, attitudes, feelings and beliefs. However, they can have an impact on the expression or performance of care. Although these factors may be difficult to measure they can be influenced by committed senior staff, good role models and good teamwork within an operating department.

Despite in some instances being difficult to measure, attempts must be made to try and assess quality in order to assure that it is being delivered. The difficulty is, of course, that quality has different elements and is often subjective. However, one excellent example of a comprehensive audit tool is the NATN QuAD which is worthy of a detailed description.

NATN QuAD

This tool follows the patient through their entire experience within the operating department and has four distinct parts.

1. Patient care
2. Departmental management
3. Patient questionnaire
4. Action plan

Patient care is further broken down into five main sections.

1. Ward/theatre department interface
2. Anaesthetic room
3. Operating room
4. Recovery room
5. Recovery room/ward interface

Each section noted above contains a number of broad standard statements which identify what is expected in terms of practice. In order to measure compliance, each standard statement has a range of questions to be asked or observations to be made which are referred to as criteria. In addition, each criterion has a data source which simply identifies where the auditor can get the information from. There are three different data sources.

1. Documentation
   - Nursing records
   - Patient charts
   - Medical and paramedical staff
2. Observation
   - Individual practitioners
   - Environment
3. Questioning
   - Direct (face to face) with patients and practitioners
   - Indirect (questionnaire) with patients and practitioners

The criteria are set out to receive a specific response: Yes (complete), Yes (incomplete), No and Not Applicable (N/A). The collated responses are then scored to provide a quantitative result.

Yes (complete)	=	*1*
Yes (incomplete)	=	*1/2*
No	=	*0*
N/A	=	*X*

The total score as a percentage is then calculated using the following formula:

$$\frac{\text{Total number of Yes}}{\text{Total applicable questions}} \times 100 = [\text{SCORE}]$$

(N/A responses are not included in the final calculation.)

The qualitative result is achieved by collating free text comments made by the auditor.

Sections within the document are also left blank so that local standards can be defined and measured in the same format. Figure 5.2 sets out the example from the NATN QuAD tool.

The patient is transported to and is safely cared for in the reception area

EXAMPLE

Data source	Criteria	Comments
Observe	The ward nurse conducts a preoperative check prior to the patient leaving (must include: Name band; Removal of jewellery; Removal of prosthesis; Signed consent form)	

	1	2	3	4	5	6	7	8	9	10
Yes C	✓	✓	✓			✓				
Yes I				✓	✓			✓	✓	
No							✓			✓
N/A										
Score	1	1	1	1/2	1/2	1	0	1/2	1/2	0

PT 4 No Name band check

PT 5 No Name band check

PT 8 No consent form check

PT 9 No Name band check

Example

$$\frac{(4 \times 1) + (4 \times 1/2)}{10} = \frac{4 + 2}{10} \times \frac{100}{1} = 60\%$$

Figure 5.2 The ward/operating department interface.

The critical part, as with any research or audit project, is what you do with the information gleaned. It needs to be disseminated throughout the department and an action plan identified for the issues that need to be addressed. A named individual must be given the responsibility for dealing with the issue and a time frame set with a review date to ensure that action has been taken.

Developing quality assurance

Auditing quality gives very useful information that can help in developing quality standards and programmes. Quality programmes need to be both 'top down', with the commitment and leadership of senior staff, and 'bottom up', with the enthusiasm and expertise of all staff to take ownership of the processes.

There also needs to be an understanding of what quality assurance is for. Quality care needs to become the focus of every activity undertaken in the operating theatre. In order to help nurses focus on their individual performance and the effectiveness of that performance, each practitioner must continually ask the following questions.

- Why do we do what we do?
- How do we know that what we do works?
- How can we improve what we do?
- How do we know we have improved?

Quality assurance is achieved through quality assessment with subsequent action leading to quality improvement. It is essentially based on set standards that are either statutory or agreed by experts in a specified field. Regular audits are undertaken to ensure that the standards are being achieved with the assumption that if they have been correctly defined and reviewed, a high quality of service will follow.

The RCN (1990) developed the Dynamic Standard Setting System (DYSSY) which encouraged local groups of nurses to determine their own standards for their ward's or department's work. At that time it was nurses generally dealing with nursing matters whereas more recently the drive has been to adopt a more multidisciplinary approach focusing on the patient's needs. Many perioperative nurses adopted this approach and found one of its main drawbacks was the amount of time involved in writing the standards, trying to agree words and nuances because of personal or professional considerations.

All this is very time consuming, so there are benefits in being able to access tools that set out predetermined standards and a framework for auditing those standards. These have been developed nationally and can be bought 'off the shelf'. The two tools that offer this approach for use within an operating theatre environment are the NATN QuAD (as described in detail above) and the King's Fund Organisational Audit (1991). Both of these documents have explicit standards and a measurement tool which serves to assess compliance of the operating department with these standards.

Making quality work

It can be seen that improving quality requires a multifaceted approach. In simple terms, there are four core aspects – plan, do, check, act.

Box 5.2 maps out the key elements of a quality strategy, based on an approach adopted in Potter et al (1994). The successful implementation of a quality strategy will depend on addressing each of these issues.

Box 5.2 Key elements of a quality strategy (based on Potter et al 1994)

Quality assurance	*Organisational culture*
Standard setting	Training
Clinical audit	Communication networks
Risk management	Policies and procedures
Review mechanisms, e.g. QuAD	Staff ownership
	Leadership
Patient information	*Monitoring processes*
Questionnaires	Clinical indicators
Focus groups	Record keeping
Postoperative visits	Performance indicators
Complaints procedures	Benchmarking

CONCLUSION

This chapter has illustrated how health-care providers try to ensure that they provide a quality service. It is recognised that quality is a difficult concept to pin down and measure, but every effort must be made to continuously improve quality. Today's perioperative nurses need to be able to continuously audit, evaluate and assure the quality of care they provide, ensuring that it is underpinned wherever possible with evidence-based practice. 'Sacred cows', practice that is carried out because 'it's always been done that way', must be things of the past. This is not because the practice is necessarily bad but because practice must be reviewed and changed where appropriate to reflect what is determined through research and audit to be best practice. This in turn will ensure a high quality of care for patients.

REFERENCES

Department of Health 1997a The new NHS: modern, dependable. Stationery Office, London
Department of Health, Scottish Office 1997b Designed to care: renewing the National Health Service in Scotland. Stationery Office, Edinburgh
Department of Health, Welsh Office 1997c Putting patients first: the future of the NHS in Wales. Stationery Office, Cardiff
King's Fund 1991 Organisational audit. King Edward's Hospital Fund, London

Long A, Harrison S 1996 The balance of evidence. Health Service Journal, Health Management Guide Issue Number 6: 1–2

McClarey M, Duff L 1997 Clinical effectiveness and evidence-based practice. Nursing Standard 11(52): 33–37

National Association of Theatre Nurses 1994 Quality assessment document (QuAD). NATN, Harrogate

NHS Executive 1996 Promoting clinical effectiveness: a framework for action in and through the NHS. DoH, London

Ovretveit J 1996 Health service quality, 2nd edn. Blackwell Science, Oxford

Potter C, Morgan P, Thompson A 1994 Continuous quality improvement in an acute hospital. International Journal of Healthcare Quality Assurance 7(1): 4–29

RCN 1990 Quality patient care: the dynamic standard setting system. Scutari, Harrow

RCN 1996 The RCN clinical effectiveness initiative: a strategic framework. RCN, London

Smith C 1997 Evidence based nursing. Nursing Management 3(10): 22–23

White S J 1997 Evidence based practice and nursing: the new panacea? British Journal of Nursing 6(3): 175–178

Williams M 1994 The trouble with quality. British Journal of Theatre Nursing 4(7): 11–12

FURTHER READING

Evidence-based nursing – linking research to practice. RCN Publishing Company and the BMJ Publishing Group. Journal web site: http://www.evidencebasenursing.com

National Association of Theatre Nurses 1994 Quality assessment document (QuAD). NATN, Harrogate

Ovretveit J 1996 Health service quality, 2nd edn. Blackwell Science, Oxford

USEFUL ADDRESSES

National Association of Theatre Nurses
Daisy Ayris House
6 Grove Park Court
Harrogate HG1 4DP
Phone: 01423 508079
e-mail: hq@natn.org.uk
website: www.natn.org.uk

Perioperative risk management

Jo Wilson

The area of perioperative practice has long been the focus of risk management concerns. Providing perioperative care is a risky business, which is heavily reliant on having appropriate staff with the right skills and competency levels, clear policies, procedures and clinical guidelines and effective teamwork to oversee the continuity of care issues. Patient and staff safety is paramount in this highly technical, specialised area and continuously improving the quality of care is essential and can be achieved by having a proactive clinical risk management system which protects all parties and the environment by assessing, identifying, controlling, minimising and evaluating risks.

A clinical risk strategy supported by a localised manual with clear procedures and policies for people, equipment, materials, hazardous substances, moving and handling and sterilisation safety is a must. The National Association of Theatre Nurses *Risk assessment guide* (NATN 1996) is an excellent tool for workplace risk assessments and for guiding staff towards action planning for evaluating risks or hazards in the theatre area. This guide should be used in conjunction with and to inform developments in the operative department's clinical risk strategy and manual. A designated person should take the lead for risk coordination with the proviso that risk management is a process, not a position, and as such it is part of every person's role and responsibility. Teamwork is a necessary ingredient to ensure all staff are caring for each other's and patient safety.

Adverse patient outcomes and communication failures are most frequently caused by a breakdown in the continuity of care as the patient moves through the operating department. At least 25% of all clinical incidents occur in the intraoperative period. Many of these incidents relate to negligent administration of anaesthesia or the negligent - monitoring of patients under anaesthesia. The effective management of clinical risk of liability exposures requires a coordinated, integrated perioperative process which focuses on providing safe, high-quality patient care.

The whole arena of perioperative care incorporating all aspects of day surgery and minor surgery undertaken by GPs can be hazardous if the appropriate controls and checking mechanisms are not in place. Any kind of surgical intervention is likely to take place in a highly technical area further complicated by the size of the perioperative team and the intricacies of equipment. During an operation requiring general anaesthesia, a patient is generally sedated, paralysed, intubated and placed on mechanical equipment that assumes the breathing function. Unconscious or heavily sedated patients rarely cause their own injuries, making each team member responsible for becoming the patient's advocate. Due to these complexities the potential for error and liability is high, therefore making it essential that staff are always trying to prevent negligent behaviour, enhancing communication and supported by accurate documentation.

The principles of risk management can be applied practically to all of these areas with specific emphasis on:

- agreement and consent and the information supplied about the procedure;
- preparation of the patient including the importance of communication;
- patient identification and the checking processes;
- patient monitoring through all aspects of perioperative care;
- patient positioning and movement within the operating theatre environment;
- familiarisation, maintenance and usage of equipment;
- the importance of perioperative procedures throughout the continuum of care.

The emphasis will be on raising risk awareness; changing, monitoring and evaluating practice; risk modification of clinical behaviour and ensuring defensibility through stringent controls if and when things do go wrong; and providing support to practitioners when things do go wrong.

CLINICAL RISK MANAGEMENT STRATEGY

Clinical risk management (CRM) addresses the synergy between risk management, quality and the legal system (Table 6.1). Risk management can be defined as the systematic identification, assessment and reduction of risks to patients and staff and the prevention and avoidance of untoward incidences and events. Quality is all about providing optimal care through controlled processes using policies, procedures, guidelines and multidisciplinary standards that are measured, monitored and evaluated by the perioperative team.

The legal issues may focus on the removal of Crown immunity and the introduction of Crown indemnity from January 1990. This led to trusts managing their own liability on health-care legislation for professional liability, health and safety at work, safe systems of work and COSHH, etc., all of which have an impact on perioperative nurses.

Table 6.1 Clinical risk management

Risk management	Quality assurance
Legally acceptable care with the identification of risks which have an adverse effect on the quality, safety and effectiveness of care delivery.	Optimal patient care demonstrated through the use of evidence-based practice and clinical effectiveness.
Data collection and chart review identifies risks, assessment and evaluation of those risks and positive action to eliminate or reduce them.	Audit/peer review identifies problems and provides the forum for discussion of benchmarking good practices.
Focuses on reducing legal costs and settlements and repairing the system breakdowns.	Focuses on improving patient care and meeting reasonable standards of practice.
Concentrates on claims prevention and management and learning the lessons for safer and more effective systems of care.	Reduction in claims is seen as a byproduct and analysis of claims allows tightening up of processes through policies, procedures and clinical guideline updating.

Important areas to address

● *Awareness and evaluation* – including assessment of the present situation, identification of potential and actual risk with analysis and evaluation. Risk awareness and risk identification is the first part of the CRM strategy.

● *Education and implementation* – including control of the risks by assigning responsibility for avoidance, including ways of minimising or eliminating risk exposure or ways of dealing with risk acceptance with planned coordination and prevention. This has to allow for risk taking, which should not be discouraged in order to facilitate innovations, research and developments.

● *Integration and support* – having a reporting mechanism with a coordinated incident and occurrence tracking system where staff feel supported rather than threatened in reporting events. This requires an open, honest and 'blame-free' culture where staff are prepared to report and learn from situations in order to improve processes and systems of care delivery.

Any CRM strategy requires a strong commitment to education, accountability and communication. In the operating department in particular, staff must feel part of a valued team of professionals with responsibility for the safety and quality of patient care. To support the strategy, there are many guidance documents and supporting literature such as:

● *Quality assessment document* (NATN 1994);
● *Risk assessment guide* (NATN 1996);
● *Principles of safe practice in the perioperative environment* (NATN 1998a);
● *Safeguards for invasive procedures* (NATN 1998b);
● *MDU theatre safeguards, informed consent, anaesthetic risks and day unit surgery;*

- *National and local standards and charters;*
- *Code of Professional Conduct* (UKCC 1992).

Perioperative staff need to be applying these tools and checklists in order to monitor their systems and measure for continuous quality improvements.

Risk occurrence areas in the operating department

- Wrong patient
- Anaesthetic awareness
- Retained swabs, needles, instruments, drill pieces – incorrect counts
- Instrument breakage
- Wrong operation
- Wrong operation site
- Incorrect positioning of patients – postoperative nerve damage
- Falls off theatre trolley/table
- No written consent/lack of informed consent
- Unplanned surgery not covered by the consent
- Patient burns resulting from equipment
- Tourniquet injuries
- Unplanned disconnection from equipment that has the potential for patient injury
- Potential contamination from break in sterile technique
- Cardiac and/or respiratory arrest during surgery
- Undertaking additional procedures which have not been given consent
- Staff working beyond their skills and competency levels
- Lack of supervision for junior staff
- Inadequate preoperative work-up with investigations/X-rays not being undertaken or results not available

These occurrences and more plague the perioperative team players in what is already a stressful scenario requiring total concentration and split-second judgement. Some of these will now be discussed to help practitioners understand their liabilities that often arise when a patient alleges malpractice in the operating department.

Communication and documentation

From a prevention aspect, there is no greater shield than an effective communication strategy supported by adequate documentation with efficient, conscientious communication between the patient and the team. This issue is intensified by the need for the patient's consent to the procedures to be performed, procedures most often obscure to the patient and within the control of the operating department staff. There is a need for constant awareness and full and accurate communication and documentation for a smooth process to minimise risks to patients and staff. Clear and complete documentation of all processes is the best form of defence if and when things go wrong. Intraoperative care plans or *multidisciplinary pathways of care*© (Wilson 1992) are effective risk management tools.

Informed consent

Informed consent is a legal concept which requires that before agreeing to a procedure or treatment, patients or their legal guardians be advised of and understand:

- the risks, benefits and alternatives;
- the risks and benefits of not following the recommended treatment plan;
- expected postoperative lifestyle/health status;
- likelihood of blood transfusion;
- involvement of junior doctors in the procedure and the presence of outside observers.

This is echoed in the Patient's Charter (1992): 'Patients are to be given a clear explanation of any treatment proposed, including risks and alternatives, before they decide whether they will agree to treatment'. Ideally informed consent should be obtained by the person undertaking the procedure who has the best knowledge to offer full explanation to the patient.

The informed consent decision-making process is complex, ideally beginning with the first encounter with the patient. It is an ongoing process that invites patients to be full partners in their own care. This should be signed and documented in the patient's record and supported by adequate information leaflets to enhance the patient's understanding and allow time for questions or point of clarification. Discussions should also take place around the issue of autologous blood transfusion. This process provides the patient with the option of refusing or declining a proposed treatment or procedure, basing that decision on sufficient information to acknowledge the potential outcome.

It is difficult to believe that when the medical staff go beyond the level of the procedure consented for, the nurses and ODPs are not aware or do not feel they have a duty of care to ensure that the patient is informed and/or the appropriate procedures have been documented. In a number of cases which have gone through or are going through the legal process, the nurses and ODPs have not always acted as the patient's advocate for fear of undermining the medical staff. These have included 'open and shut cases' where patients have not been informed of their condition/prognosis; cases of ovaries being removed and HRT being inserted and hysterectomies being performed during caesarean sections on histologically normal uteruses and without good clinical indications. The operating department team must be aware of what has been consented for and if the procedure goes beyond this, should ensure the patient is informed and the total procedure is documented in the patient records.

Patient identification

Identification of the patient should be undertaken by the ward nurse, reception nurse, anaesthetist, perioperative nurse and surgeon by checking the patient name and identification bracelet, the side, site and name of the proposed operative procedure. This is undertaken by the following methods:

- Asking the patient.
- Checking the patient identification bracelet.
- Reviewing the patient records and comparing the data with the operating list.
- Completing the checklist and ensuring completeness of patient records and X-rays for procedure being undertaken.

Patient monitoring – recommended minimum

There are minimum recommendations for all patients undergoing a procedure requiring a general or regional anaesthesia, including having a qualified anaesthetist present at all times. The following baseline observations are the recommended minimum.

- Blood pressure (systolic/diastolic or mean arterial BP)
- Pulse
- ECG pattern and heart rate
- Precordial or oesophageal breath/heart sounds
- Pulse oximetry
- Temperature – for all paediatric cases and all adult cases lasting longer than 30 minutes

Patient positioning and movement

Care should be taken when positioning or moving unconscious patients in theatre. Documentation of each patient's position and precautions taken to prevent positional injury is the individual and collective responsibility of the members of the perioperative team. Due consideration should be given to the following:

- Avoidance of peripheral nerve injuries.
- Avoidance of other mechanical trauma.
- Mechanical interference with cardiovascular or respiratory function.
- Positioning and placement of instruments, diathermy and heat-related appliances.
- Illumination and exposure to ensure ability to assess the patient's colour.

Tied into this is the importance of moving and handling training for all staff for their own and patient safety. This should include all grades and disciplines of staff who are involved in moving patients, equipment or instrument trays. So often, the TSSU/CSSD staff have no manual handling training and they often lift and move heavy loads continuously. Systems should be put in place to minimise lifting by sliding or automating the process of moving heavy trays and instruments.

Accountable items

There should be established policies, procedures and guidelines concerning instrument, swab and needle counts, including appropriate documentation. Practitioners should not allow outside distractions to interfere with their duty to report correct counts. Maintaining the same staff during a procedure helps to ensure continuity and safety. Changing of staff should be kept to a minimum.

The count should be undertaken before the procedure starts, following the surgery and prior to skin closure and at the end of the procedure. The operator should be informed immediately if the count is incorrect and the appropriate action should be taken.

Members of staff can be held liable for incorrect counts even if the surgeon has overall responsibility and delegates the task of counting (Case study 6.1). This area of accountability is not completely clear; the following American case illustrates that each case is judged on an individual basis and that the law is not black and white.

Case study 6.1   Ravi v Williams (1988)

In 1988 in the USA a surgeon was accused of leaving a sponge in a patient's abdomen. The surgeon's defence was that he had delegated the responsibility of the sponge count to the nurses and they negligently told him the count was correct so he felt he was absolved from further responsibility.

The Alabama Supreme Court disagreed; they stated the surgeon alone has the responsibility for removing all sponges. The nurses' responsibility for counting the sponges after removal is only an added precaution taken by the surgeon to help ensure that he has properly performed his duty.

The act of leaving swabs in a patient raises a strong suggestion of negligence and the claimant's solicitors do not need to produce expert testimonies to prove that the act falls below the standard of care required by surgeons. This is an area where team play is essential and staff need to meticulously follow policies, procedures and documentation of counts. In so many cases, when investigations begin, the team remember the count was correct but there is a lack of documentation and the evidence speaks for itself.

Surgical equipment

Advances in technology continue to produce more sophisticated and more expensive equipment. To effectively address the potential exposures related to the uses and abuses of all equipment used in the operating department, a monitoring tracking method system with quality review indicators needs to be used continually. All safety checks and infection control measures need to be documented, including all initial and ongoing checks on the safety aspects and use of the equipment. All equipment should meet the current standards and be adequate to provide safe services to patients. When equipment fails or malfunctions it should be taken out of use and labelled and not used again until all investigation, safety and maintenance checks are undertaken. All maintenance and repair records should be documented and reviewed periodically to identify trends. Back-up equipment should be available where necessary.

Operating department staff should only be allowed to use equipment if they have the requisite skills, expertise and competencies. New equipment or trial equipment should be adequately demonstrated and staff should be familiar with its usage before it is used on patients. A record should be maintained to demonstrate appropriate training and regular updates on usage and maintenance. Trying out new equipment directly on patients, with sales representatives present, is not safe practice.

CLINICAL GOVERNANCE

In the 1997 White Paper *The new NHS: modern, dependable* (DoH 1997), the systems of clinical governance mark a fundamental and significant shift towards involving clinicians in the assurance of both quality and accountability in health-care delivery. The paper states: 'The government will require every NHS trust to embrace the concept of clinical governance, so that quality is at the core, both of their responsibilities as organisations and of each of their staff as individual professionals'. In order to achieve this, the government will bring forward legislation to give NHS trusts a new duty to take responsibility for the quality of care and working in partnership across health and social care. Under these arrangements, chief executives will carry ultimate responsibility for assuring the quality of the services provided by their trust, just as they are already accountable for the proper use of resources.

In *A first class service: quality in the NHS* (DoH 1998), clinical governance is:

> . . . *defined as a framework through which the NHS organisations are accountable for continuously improving the quality of their services and safeguarding high standards of care by creating an environment in which excellence in clinical care will flourish.*

The principles of clinical governance apply to all those who provide or manage patient care services in the NHS. It requires staff to work in partnership providing integrated care (Wilson 1996) within health and social care teams, between practitioners and managers and between the NHS, patients and the public.

Principles of clinical governance

Clinical governance incorporates a number of processes, including:

- clinical audit;
- evidence-based practice in daily use supported within the infrastructure;

- clinical effectiveness;
- clinical risk management with adverse events being detected, openly investigated and lessons learned;
- lessons for improving practice are learned from complaints;
- outcomes of care;
- good-quality clinical data to monitor clinical care with problems of poor clinical practice being recognised early and dealt with;
- good practice systematically disseminated within and outside the organisation;
- clinical risk reduction programmes of a high standard in place.

Clinical governance places a duty of responsibility on all health-care professionals to ensure that care is satisfactory, consistent and responsive. Each individual will be responsible for the quality of their clinical practice as part of professional self-regulation.

Clinical governance processes

The following steps must be taken to ensure that proper performance measures and responsibilities are being taken to assure the quality of care.

- Clinical quality improvements integrated with the overall organisational continuous quality improvement programmes.
- Good practice systematically disseminated.
- Clinical risk reduction programmes in place.
- Professional self-regulation/assessment including the development of clinical leadership skills.
- Evidence-based practice systems in place.
- Adverse events, near misses and incidents detected, openly investigated and lessons learned.
- Complaints dealt with positively and the information used to improve the organisation and care delivery.
- High-quality performance measurement data collected to monitor clinical care.
- Poor clinical performance dealt with appropriately to minimise harm to patients and other staff.
- Continuing professional development aligned with clinical governance principles.

All these issues need to be addressed and incorporated for all grades and disciplines of staff within the operating department risk management documentation.

Dimensions of clinical governance

There are three dimensions to clinical governance.

1. *Corporate accountability* for clinical performance with the chief executive/chair of governing body with overall responsibility – the

'accountable officer' role. There may be a board subcommittee led by a clinical professional such as the medical director or chief nurse, expected to provide monthly reports to the board and arrangements in the annual report.

2. *Internal mechanisms* for improving clinical performance including individual accountability, self and professional regulation.

3. *External mechanisms* for improving clinical performance – Commission for Health Improvement (CHIMP), 'the watchdog with a smile and sharp teeth'. CHIMP is a statutory body to support those who are developing and monitoring local systems and multidisciplinary standards for clinical quality. It offers an independent guarantee that local systems to monitor, assure and improve clinical quality are in place. It also has the capacity to offer specific support on request when local organisations face particular clinical problems. It also investigates and identifies the sources of problems and works with organisations on lasting remedies to improve quality and standards of patient care.

These three dimensions ensure there are proper processes in place for continually monitoring and improving clinical quality and enhancing patient and staff safety within the operating theatre suite. Every health-care organisation has a clinical professional to take charge of quality issues and there is a legal duty of quality imposed on every organisation. CHIMP works with and helps organisations to develop quality criteria, monitoring, measurement and evaluation as well as policing the adoption and operation of clinical governance.

Quality of care is everybody's business

In Walshe (1998), Frank Dobson (the then Health Secretary) was quoted as saying:

> We've got to raise standards in the NHS. We've also got to make the NHS more helpful and responsive to patients when things go wrong so fewer people will feel the need to turn to the lawyers. We want explanation, not litigation. Apologies, not accusations. Excellence, not excuses.

In order to raise standards, there needs to be a comprehensive clinical benchmarking system across the NHS, which will include perioperative care, to compare and share best practices. There is no point in every health-care organisation reinventing the wheel and all going in different directions in order to achieve the same agenda. The National Institute of Clinical Excellence (NICE) will promote the use of clinical guidelines derived from evidence-based practice with inbuilt advice on clinical audit criteria and evaluation. It will have a role in the assessment of prime research and systematic reviews and appraisal of clinical guidelines. This new centre, which will be accountable to the Health Secretary for its resources, work programme and for the guidance it produces for the NHS, will provide information on clinical and cost effectiveness and sharing of best practices.

HEALTH-CARE PERFORMANCE MEASUREMENTS

In the past, attempts to measure clinical performance and the usage of clinical indicators have been actively resisted by the medical profession. Obstacles such as the difficulty of collecting data, problems in gaining compliance, confidentiality concerns and the difficulties of comparing like with like have been constantly put forward. Even the Patient's Charter, launched 8 years ago, carefully restricted itself to waiting times, waiting lists and administrative measures.

Within the medical profession, progressive pioneers were pushing doctors to be more open. Brendan Devlin at the Royal College of Surgeons introduced the *Confidential enquiry into perioperative deaths* (CEPOD), a series of audits on crucial operations, but was forced to keep them confidential and informal. Up to 30% of surgeons and anaesthetists have not participated in CEPOD and problems with confidentiality have enabled some of the worst examples of hazards to patients to be brushed aside. The *Confidential enquiry into maternal mortality* (CEMM) and the *Confidential enquiry into stillbirths and deaths in infancy* (CESDI) have achieved higher levels of participation but still their confidential and informal nature has enabled some practitioners to ignore the recommendations. In 1997 Dr Anthony Hopkins, director of the Royal College of Physicians, publicly damned audits for their poor standards and called for much clearer lines of accountability. The USA had open audit years ago, but the UK remained sceptical. This became more difficult to sustain with the successful introduction of audit in Scotland and the Scottish Office *Review of acute services*, which have already helped to raise standards.

In Frank Dobson's words: 'We need a system which collects and monitors information on clinical performance, provides an early warning if things are going wrong, and then helps put things right' (*Guardian*, June 11 1998). There is one scandal which made audit possible: the Bristol Royal Infirmary doctors who continued to operate on babies long after they should have stopped. Britain's biggest ever medical disciplinary inquiry, which concluded in May 1998, found one Bristol doctor had a mortality rate of 60% for hole in the heart operations when the national average was 14% while another, performing an arterial switch procedure, had a two in three death rate when the national average was one in 10. In 59 operations, 29 babies died and four more were brain damaged. Other recent failures such as those at the Devon and Exeter and the Kent and Canterbury hospitals have pushed clinical governance to the top of the health-care agenda. Even the BMA called for the collection of death rates, readmission and re-operation rates to prevent another 'Bristol'. Even more surprising, leading members of the medical profession have welcomed the move.

Experiences in perioperative performance measurement in the USA

MMI Companies Inc, a health-care risk management company based in Chicago, have consistently analysed clinical practice, quality of care, patient outcomes and clinical negligence data to gain a clear understanding of the human, organisational and environmental factors that correlate with adverse patient outcomes. This ongoing data analysis is anchored to their risk-claims link process. It encompasses a continuous review of clinical negligence claims in the context of the MMI clinical risk modification programmes, along with the evaluation of clinical practice and outcomes data through an approved Joint Commission on Accreditation of Healthcare Organisations (JCAHO) accepted clinical indicators programme. The cornerstone of this successful data collection, which has recently been updated into a *12-year data summary resource* (MMI 1998), is an array of clinical risk management strategies and sharing of experiences and resources. These have been supported by the MMI risk modification triad of information, consultation and education, which helps health-care providers to demonstrate that they can achieve excellence to reduce the risk of adverse outcomes (Fig. 6.1).

The risk modification programmes are developed by multidisciplinary teams of health-care professionals and combine clinical guidelines, clinical indicators and patient record review criteria in an effort to help providers focus on improving systems and practices to decrease the risk of injury. Healthcare Risk Resources International (HRRI, a UK-based health-care risk management company), through its clinical advisory group, has been reviewing the MMI programmes and undertaking a closed claims analysis of UK claims which demonstrates a high level of comparability between the USA and UK clinical negligence systems. The important factor for the UK system is the emphasis on volume, practice and outcomes measures to ensure the comparing of like with like and to

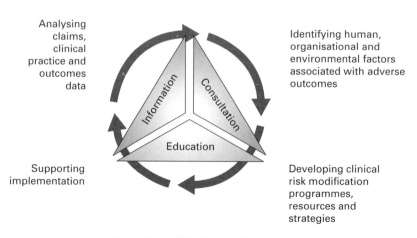

Figure 6.1 MMI risk modification triad.

facilitate the root cause of analysis errors. Each clinical indicator includes purpose, data elements, data sources, definitions, rate calculation, diagram of indicator relationship and applicable record review criteria.

MMI's programmes have helped health-care organisations not only control costs but also improve quality of care. Previous data collected from participating hospitals showed that the use of pulse oximetry appeared to correlate with fewer anaesthesia-related complications during surgery. Pulse oximetry is a non-invasive monitoring technology that assesses oxygen levels in the blood. With the increasing prevalence of the newer intravenous conscious sedation technique used across clinical settings, MMI began aggressively encouraging the use of pulse oximetry with this type of anaesthesia across all settings. Over a 3-year period, from 1994 to 1996, the percentage of cases in which this monitoring technology was used with intravenous conscious sedation increased among participating organisations by as much as 84%. Given the benefits noted with this practice, increased awareness and compliance help enhance patient safety in those settings.

With more and more patients receiving care in day care settings, it is essential that monitoring practices that reduce risk to inpatients move with patients to alternative sites of care. At a time when there is a national focus on patient safety, these findings help our health-care providers identify and change patterns of care that put patients at risk of injury. Another area that confirms the distinct connection between clinical practice and patient outcomes emerges from the surgical guidelines. The data suggest that health-care providers are doing an effective job of selecting appropriate clinical settings and surgical techniques for patients by the effective use of patient evaluation and selection criteria. This correlates with a low rate of unplanned returns to surgery within 48 hours, as well as a low rate of injuries to organs resulting from the use of an endoscope during surgery (in each case, rates are less than 1%).

MMI and HRRI's goals are to help health-care providers to take a more systematic approach to clinical practice in order to improve patient outcomes. By identifying their potential risk exposures, health-care organisations can work to modify those risks, with a particular emphasis on applying risk modification programmes to improve patient safety and health-care quality. The collection of data helps to provide health-care organisations with the insight necessary to achieve these goals.

DATA COLLECTION IN HEALTH-CARE ORGANISATIONS

Health-care organisations in all sectors of care delivery need to demonstrate their high levels of achievement and commitment to continuous quality improvements. Risk management is a process for the identification of risks which have adverse effects on the quality, safety and effectiveness of service delivery, the assessment and evaluation of those risks and for the initiation of positive action to eliminate or reduce them. Having an open, honest and blame-free organisation which is open to improving processes and systems of care is a big step towards having staff committed to quality and getting things right. Near miss, incident and indicator recording and reporting are cornerstones to any quality and risk management system.

Incident reporting, investigation and follow-up are considered a minimum, level one standard of the *Clinical Negligence Scheme for Trusts* (Wilson 1998a) alongside the clinical complaints procedure as a means of assessing areas where improvements need to be made. The reporting of near misses is also important as we can learn from these and put systems in place to stop them happening. A definition of a near miss may be 'an occurrence which but for luck or skilful management would in all probability have become an incident' (Wilson 1998b). As health-care professionals, we need to be prepared to share things that have the potential to go wrong and to have a learning culture to prevent patient accident or injuries occurring in the first place.

A clinical incident may be defined as 'any occurrence which is not consistent with the professional standards of care of the patient or the routine operation/policies of the organisation' (Wilson 1998b). Experience to date shows that a 1000-bed NHS trust with a bed occupancy of 89% can expect to have 5800 clinical incidents, of which 116 have the potential for some form of compensation and around 38 of which could become clinical negligence claims. None of us gets out of bed in the morning and deliberately sets out to harm or injure any patient yet we all know that in dealing with people, it is inevitable that some accidents/incidents do occur. Collection of near miss and clinical incident data is essential in perioperative care to ensure mistakes are rectified, lessons are learned and practices are modified to reduce risks. Some of the pitfalls and failings of the common systems are:

- due to some activities being given low priority, the failure of staff to identify serious events;
- the fear of reporting perceptions with finger pointing and blame being applied instead of support and help to put things right;
- punitive response, especially for some disciplines such as nursing where many incidents result in disciplinary action;
- having the wrong systems or inadequate policies, procedures and guidelines in the first place.

Each health-care organisation should have a clear definition of clinical incidents. They should encourage reporting without the threat of punitive responses and speciality-specific as well as organisation-wide examples of what constitutes a near miss and incident should serve as a guide. Many health-care organisations have undertaken this with the support of a letter to every member of staff from the chief executive reinforcing an open and honest culture and highlighting that no member of staff will be disciplined unless an incident was malicious, criminal, kept recurring without lessons being learned or constituted gross professional misconduct.

It is extremely important that near misses and incidents are tracked and trended to provide information to support the lessons which need to be learned, inform the education and training programmes and revised policies, procedures and guidelines, building on the strengths of where things go right and analysing and improving the areas of weaknesses. Recording of incident information within a database and investigating events in a timely manner allow appropriate action to be set within a clear time frame to limit damages and prevent recurrences through reviewing practices and procedures and providing feedback to staff.

The areas where incidents occur focus around places where patients pass through the health-care system, such as the operating department, and are reliant on good communication and documentation. The perioperative period is a particularly difficult time in these respects, due to the fact that patients are sedated or anaesthetised and have to rely on staff being their advocate with adequate checks to ensure the right patient is in the right place at the right time and having the correct procedure. Clinical indicators which are speciality-specific triggers or early warning signs of things which need further review or investigation are an important component of clinical incident recording. These clinical indicators are based on the analysis of clinical negligence claims, which identify common activities where things do go wrong. They provide the following.

- 'Top of the trees' triggers which look at events that serve as a flag for deeper review through the clinical audit and effectiveness processes.

- Timely comparative data source with potential benchmarking opportunities with other specialities in other trusts on a national basis to allow sharing and implementation of best practices and lessons learned.

- Triggers to drive decision making and promote behaviour change as necessary, which is one of the most important components of risk management. If behaviour and practices do not change then accidents and litigation will continue to be a drain on health-care resources.

The anaesthetic clinical practice indicators (see Box 6.1), which have been monitored over the last 12 years, include the following.

- Non-emergency general anaesthesia without documented preanaesthesia airway evaluation.
- General/regional anaesthesia cases – continuous pulse oximetry not used in immediate recovery period.
- Regional analgesia/anaesthesia without continuous pulse oximetry.
- Intravenous conscious sedation without continuous pulse oximetry.

Box 6.1 Most common serious incidents in anaesthetics

- Breathing circuit disconnections
- Inadequate gas flows
- Syringe swap
- Gas supply problems
- Anaesthetic awareness
- Hypovolaemia
- Problems with endotracheal tube
- Disconnected intravenous lines
- Circuit misconnection
- Wrongly connected tubing or modified vaporisers
- Malfunction of laryngoscope
- Premature extubation

The clinical outcome indicators have been based on the following criteria.

- Cases cancelled due to difficult intubation.
- Intraprocedural deaths or cardiopulmonary arrests.
- Deaths or cardiopulmonary arrests during the immediate recovery period.
- Deaths/arrests within 48 hours of anaesthesia administration.
- Deaths/arrests within 48 hours of intravenous conscious sedation.
- Central nervous system deficits within 48 hours of anaesthesia administration.
- Unplanned inpatient admissions within 48 hours of outpatient/day surgery.

Effective near miss, clinical incident and indicator/trigger systems can provide essential information for education and development of staff; improvements in the health-care organisation documentation for improving clinical practice; early identification of potential risk of clinical negligence cases, including the provision of details such as statements from staff involved and location of their whereabouts; and an estimation of defensibility, liability and early settlement of potential or actual claims against the organisation. Incident reporting, complaints and claims management need to be brought together under one umbrella to inform the risk management processes and to allow them to become more proactive than reactive, supporting the notion that prevention is cheaper than cure and certainly better for the patient in terms of quality of care.

Day-care surgery and procedures

In recent years, health care has been transformed by the shift to day care and outpatient care. Now, health-care risk management must also be transformed within this new arena of highly integrated health-care services. The principles of identification, analysis and treatment of clinical risk must be applied across multiple new settings. Risk managers who are familiar with the acute inpatient care setting and its systems for monitoring and evaluation will find an exciting challenge as they broaden their reach across all the integrated day or outpatient care services. Today's swift move by trusts to provide more care in day-case and outpatient settings is increasing the risk of clinical negligence but few directors and managers are acknowledging, managing or watching this.

When entering this new arena, it is important for risk managers to develop good relationships with clinicians by being accessible and by providing education and feedback. Implementing risk modification strategies can follow naturally after mutual interest in reducing risk and improving the delivery of quality care has been established. Some of the steps that can be taken to introduce risk management techniques in the day-care and outpatient care settings are as follows.

Provide education
Discuss risk management principles and the benefits of early identification of events that may lead to claims. Include information on how communication and attitudes affect patients' tendencies to pursue litigation. Provide clinicians with practical information on how to respond to patient complaints. Give examples of general events that should trigger them to attempt to diffuse a situation. Communication is the key: communication and collaboration between the care givers supported by effective systems and processes for care delivery and documentation, and communication with patients and their families. Lack of communication with patients and their families is usually the main reason why they make a formal complaint or begin clinical negligence proceedings. The thing they want most is an explanation of 'what has happened' or 'what is actually going on'. The focus on providing good-quality risk management is an effective communication strategy.

Identify clinical risk exposures
Encourage input from clinicians about areas they feel are high risk or that have been the source of past problems. Additional sources that can be used to supplement this dialogue include formal clinical articles, adverse occurrence screening, professional organisation clinical guidelines and clinically specific claims. Claims that relate to care rendered on an outpatient basis also should be analysed for future opportunities to improve care and prevent recurrence.

During the process of identification and assessment of clinical risk, it is important to keep the focus on identifying events in day and outpatient care that may lead to adverse outcomes. Adverse outcomes that occur after a day-case patient has been admitted as an inpatient need to be included in the process.

Coordinate data collection efforts

It is important to coordinate information sharing between the inpatient and the outpatient settings. Inpatient quality assurance programmes are often already collecting information on outcomes, such as unplanned admissions related to day-case procedures. In addition, when an untoward event occurs in the day or outpatient setting, such as contrast dye reactions in day and outpatient procedures in the radiology department, new systems may need to be developed to collect this information. Identify who will be responsible for obtaining the information. Some trusts choose to incorporate clinical risk information with their current quality management systems; others may use a telephone, trigger, incident or occurrence form or facsimile to communicate with clinical management. Regardless of the chosen method, confidentiality needs to be maintained.

Review and analyse data

Clinicians and managers should meet regularly to review the data collected and to identify clinical applications from the data. This is a good opportunity to enhance the credibility of the risk manager as a partner with clinicians in improving patient care and reducing risk. It can also provide a multidisciplinary forum to review areas for improvements.

Develop change action plans to identify opportunities for improvement

Once a trend or issue is identified through data analysis, methods to address and modify the risk need to be established. For example, a rise in admissions following outpatient surgical procedures identified by data review and analysis can be referred back to the day-case or outpatient departments for risk review and analysis. In this circumstance, the risk analysis could have suggested that the probable root cause was that the day-case or outpatient department was not receiving written preoperative patient assessment information, such as the last history and physical, prior to beginning the procedures. This was found to be limiting the surgeon's ability to anticipate undesirable outcomes, leading to postoperative inpatient admissions.

Through a joint risk management and quality improvement programme, a process could be developed to provide the necessary preoperative information to doctors in a timely and consistent manner. The use of *multidisciplinary pathways of care*© (Wilson 1992) and integrated care management (Wilson 1996) has improved the documentation, communication and continuity of care in these areas. When opportunities for improvement have been identified, the risk management or quality improvement process can be used to implement the risk reduction plan, thereby improving the quality of direct patient care delivery.

Monitor impact of efforts

When the risk reduction plan is implemented in response to an identified issue, the expected results of the efforts should be outlined. These results should be described in a measurable way and linked to an anticipated improvement in the clinical care of the patient. Regular evaluations of these results will demonstrate the impact of risk reduction efforts.

Regular evaluations also enable the risk managers/coordinators to identify when change actions plans are not effective and allow an opportunity to respond accordingly.

Developing and implementing a clinical risk management programme in day-case and outpatient care is a challenge. Attention to quality and risk has a direct relation to costs. Risk in day-case and outpatient care settings is where there is a potential for a (major) loss. Poor-quality care costs money and leads to duplication in order to correct it. The goal is to reduce risks associated with providing patient care in the diverse outpatient settings in which health care is delivered. As health care moves towards the greater use of day and outpatient care, clinical risk management needs to expand its focus.

CLINICAL RISK MANAGEMENT IN ANAESTHESIA

Through the application and discussion of a case study, a number of clinical risk issues will be applied to everyday professional practice.

Issues in the administration of anaesthetics

Although the environment in which anaesthesia is administered is usually a carefully controlled area, the anaesthetic agents and the patient's response to them can be unpredictable. Injuries sustained as a result of anaesthetic administration and anaesthesia can be serious with lifelong and costly disabilities and even death. On analysis of clinical negligence claims, the three main areas of human error in anaesthetics are dental damage, patient awareness during the anaesthetic and the patient suffering from brain damage or death.

Box 6.2   Risk management in anaesthesia

- Staffing
- Equipment
- Changes and late list submission
- Preanaesthesia – no preoperative visit
- Anaesthetic administration
- Postanaesthetia – recovery and ward
- Leadership
- Verification of qualifications and training
- Skills and competency recognition
- Anaesthetist availability during anaesthetic
- Supervision
- Documentation
- Communication

Box 6.3 Risk issues in anaesthesia

- Illegible record or alteration
- Failure to diagnose or treat intraanaesthetic complications in time
- Intubation problems (oesophageal, premature extubation, unintentional extubation)
- Failure to apply knowledge
- Breathing circuit disconnect, misconnect or leaks
- Loss of oxygen or nitrous oxide supply
- Improper administration
- Improper choice of anaesthetic
- Failure to monitor
- Equipment-related problems
- Improper positioning
- Vigilance failure
- Anaesthetist leaving the room during anaesthetic administration

---

Boxes 6.2 and 6.3 highlight the risk management areas in the preparation, organisational management, induction, education and training in anaesthesia. Many proactive risk management strategies have been developed to cover issues of both potential risk and actual risk when patients are receiving anaesthetics and while they are under anaesthesia. All policies, procedures, protocols and multidisciplinary pathways of care need to be constantly reviewed to ensure that current issues and risks are being addressed.

Case study

Many of the issues which have been introduced are discussed in the following case study scenario which highlights the importance of close observation and monitoring of patients undergoing procedures under general anaesthesia and the associated risk issues.

Case study 6.1

Mary Brennan, a 28-year-old female, was admitted for orthopaedic surgical repair to the rotator cuff of the right shoulder. The condition requiring the surgery resulted from her work activities as a punch card operator. The patient was married and had two small children.

During the course of the administration of the anaesthetic but before the surgery began, an oesophageal intubation occurred, which was unrecognised until the patient arrested. Based on the anaesthesia record and the occurrence report of the anaesthetist, the condition was undetected for some 10–20 minutes. The anaesthetist claimed to have performed a tracheal intubation prior to the patient's positioning. However, after the patient was positioned, he did nothing to make certain that the endotracheal tube was in fact still in the trachea. After the positioning of the patient and before surgery was undertaken, the anaesthetist left the head of the patient on at least two and perhaps three occasions. The anaesthetist admitted to leaving the patient to answer the telephone and at another time left the patient to tie the gown of the surgical assistant. It was also the custom of the anaesthetist to leave the operating room to clean the laryngoscope after use.

Having tied the surgical assistant's gown, the anaesthetist returned to the patient and noted that her hand was blue. The anaesthetist initially thought the blood pressure cuff was too tight, but upon removal of the draping over the patient's face, noted the face to be cyanotic. Almost simultaneously with the recognition of the cyanosis, the patient suffered a cardiac arrest and resuscitation was commenced. It took almost 7 minutes of resuscitation to cause the cardiac activity to resume.

Nine hours after the event, the anaesthetist prepared a postanaesthetic progress note in which he tried to recount the events leading to the cardiac arrest. In that note it was indicated that when he recognised the cyanosis 'on the assumption of an oesophageal intubation', he extubated the patient and began bag and mask with 100% oxygen. The patient and family formally issued a clinical negligence claim through their solicitor against the anaesthetist.

Allegations and claims issues

- Anaesthetist failed to maintain appropriate observation of the patient.
- Anaesthetist failed to use pulse oximetry to determine the oxygen level of the patient.
- Anaesthetist failed to use either a precordial or oesophageal stethoscope to monitor breath sounds.
- Anaesthetist failed to make certain the endotracheal tube was in a proper position after the patient was repositioned.

The patient suffered from hypoxic encephalopathy and has been in a coma since the date of the incident. She remains in hospital care with gastrostomy feeding and incontinence and does not appear to have an appreciation of her family or surroundings. She will require lifelong nursing care and physiotherapy. Her life expectancy is estimated to be 50 years. The case was settled before trial using a structured settlement.

Risk view

The risk manager, operating department manager and perioperative team are often responsible for investigating untoward events and identifying systems or practices that led to the undesired outcome. They need to be concerned not only with finding the answers to manage the anticipated claim but also with addressing the strengths and weaknesses in systems and practice patterns to prevent the recurrence of untoward events.

The following summarises the types of risk management issues that are apparent in the analysis of the claim that resulted from Mary Brennan's incident.

Building provider awareness   The anaesthetist involved in this case was very experienced, with over 30 years of practice. The initial intubation went very smoothly and everything appeared to be under control. When the anaesthetist returned from washing his laryngoscope and answering the telephone, he noted the cyanosis and the patient arrested. With this finding, he first assessed whether the blood pressure cuff was too tight. After he found that releasing the cuff did not improve the cyanosis, he then began to assess the airway. This delay furthered the patient's hypoxia.

The perioperative team are challenged to seek opportunities to make all staff aware of the potential problems that can result from a lack of observation of the patient and misplaced priorities. Analysis of this case and sharing the facts with the team can be an effective way to impress upon the team the potential impact of inattention. Annual review of the basic priorities in assessment of resuscitation is also necessary. The team should be encouraged to assess and audit their own practices and modify those acquired habits that may inadvertently place a patient at risk.

Checking of endotracheal intubation   The technology for checking endotracheal intubation has advanced dramatically, with identification of oxygen saturation and end-tidal CO_2 readings not only after initial intubation but also as an essential component of continuous monitoring.

Establishing the standard of care in effect at the time of the actual event is crucial to the development of an effective defence. (All standards should be dated and signed upon implementation and ongoing review.) At the time of this occurrence, the use of pulse oximetry or end-tidal CO_2 was not the standard of care. There were, however, other standards that addressed the checking of endotracheal tube intubation. In this instance, the anaesthetic medical experts were critical of the anaesthetist involved because the customary practice of checking endotracheal tube intubation was not adhered to.

The anaesthetist discussed his practice for checking proper intubation in his statement. His practice after intubation was to bag the patient and subjectively evaluate the level of resistance to the inflow of air. If he felt resistance, the tube was evaluated for replacement. Since he did not feel resistance in this case, he was confident that the tube was properly placed.

Legal perspective
The medical defence experts were not critical of the fact that an oesophageal intubation took place. They recognised that this can occur

without a deviation from the standard of care. Instead, they were critical of the fact that this was not identified and remedied in a timely fashion. They all concurred independently that this anaesthetist deviated from the standard of care in place at the time, in the following ways.

• He failed to auscultate the chest to determine the inspiration of air into the lungs as well as the natural expiration of the air. If pulse oximetry was available, it should have been used.

• He failed to remain with the patient. Leaving the head of the patient is not acceptable practice.

• He failed to maintain constant observation of the patient under anaesthesia. He should have continually assessed respiratory status, colour, circulatory status and other parameters in addition to relying on electronic monitoring devices.

Risks associated with repositioning

Patients are commonly repositioned after intubation to attain the best position for the operation to be performed. Risk issues often associated with improper positioning are related to tissue and nerve injury. As such, the perioperative team are encouraged to document the names of the staff involved in positioning, the actual position of the patient and the location of padding. In this case, however, the repositioning of the patient may have been the event that caused disruption of the endotracheal tube. The anaesthetist should assess the effect of the repositioning on the ventilation of the patient first and then the team can address the alignment and padding of extremities once they are satisfied the patient is adequately ventilated. Again, constant monitoring of the patient's status through careful assessment, observation and electronic monitoring is necessary.

Documentation

When untoward events occur, the patient's medical record is closely scrutinised. Risk managers finding minimal documentation endeavour to establish whether the team provided more care than was recorded. In this case, the care given was consistent with the care which was documented by the anaesthetist. There was no documentation of ongoing vital signs, precordial or oesophageal auscultation of breath sounds or other clinical observations. The defence of this case became difficult because the defence counsel was unable to establish how quickly the cyanosis was discovered and acted upon. The handwritten note the anaesthetist made 9 hours after the event was not specific enough to help the defence and noted that the tube was assumed to be in the oesophagus at the time of the arrest.

Aside from these specific problems, the overall documentation of this patient's care was described by the defence experts as being 'sloppy', 'haphazard' and 'smacks of inattentiveness'. The team all need to realise how not only the content of the documentation but also its appearance can be used against them. Illegible, crossed-out or poorly punctuated entries and non-documentation can lead to assumptions of poor-quality care delivery. The usefulness of the *multidisciplinary pathways of care*© (Wilson 1992) is that they incorporate all elements of preoperative care and continue beyond discharge until the episode of care is complete, thereby lessening the clinical risk exposure.

Interventions after the event

When adverse patient outcomes occur, it is important that the operative department manager and risk managers are notified promptly and that they intervene to minimise the sequelae. They should immediately begin to investigate and preserve useful evidence. The managers should assess the situation with the theatre team at the first available opportunity to assist the clinicians in addressing the family's needs. Early interactions and explanations will determine whether the hospital, the clinicians and the patient/family will be able to resolve the situation to mutual satisfaction. Risk managers may use available resources such as the patient ombudsman, the clergy and others to assist the patient and family work through their grief and anger.

In addition to addressing individual cases, managers should be tracking and trending occurrences and looking at ways of implementing continuous quality improvement, education and training to improve team practices. There should also be monitoring systems in place to audit the impact and effects of the implementation changes.

Case study summary

Proactive risk management in anaesthetics is essential for prevention and ongoing surveillance of techniques and protocols in use. The Medical Defence Union and the Association of Anaesthetists have published guidelines and advice to help to identify potential risks, patient monitoring requirements and actual risks in this area. Using the risk management process helps the team to identify practices, modify behaviour and reduce exposure to risk, thereby improving quality and reducing costs. Excellent communication and comprehensive documentation is the best prevention and cannot be overemphasised. These can be supported by adequate policies, procedures and clinical guidelines or *multidisciplinary pathways of care*© (Wilson 1992) which cover all aspects of patient care. There is a need for constant communication in an efficient and conscientious manner with the patient and the team. Bearing in mind that unconscious patients rarely cause their own injuries, they are totally reliant on the independent responsibility of the team to care and communicate for them in the operating department.

Building provider awareness in the administration of anaesthesia is the best proactive management. Emphasis is on continuity of care;

leadership and supervision; having the best skills and competency levels to care for the patient at all times; having and using appropriate equipment; adequate staffing levels; an effective communication strategy; and accurate documentation of all events, in a factual and complete manner, with ongoing audit and review of cases to assess strengths and weaknesses and the potential for risk exposure and improvements.

CONCLUSION

Often when things do go wrong in the operating department they are usually due to a breakdown in the care delivery process. Staff have not followed established policies and procedures, shortcuts were taken due to staff shortages or staff followed custom and practice and did not bother to question. We are all accountable and responsible for our clinical practice which should be based upon research and clinical effectiveness. An open and honest system of care will ensure lessons are learned, practices are changed and staff can trust and support each other through all eventualities. The perioperative nursing staff operate in a multidisciplinary team and are accountable also to the other team members for their performance. Nurses are also morally accountable to their patients and their families; they should act as the patient's advocate to ensure safe standards of care. They are also employed and therefore accountable to their employer and compliance is also expected with the UKCC *Code of professional conduct* (UKCC 1992).

Distillation of 'best practice' from dubious consensus is risky, especially where accountabilities are diverse and may conflict. Remember the words of Mark Twain: 'Whenever you find yourself on the side of the majority it is time to stop and reflect'. We all have a duty to provide the best and safest care to patients and active clinical risk management is essential.

REFERENCES

Department of Health 1992 The patient's charter and you. NHS Executive, Leeds
Department of Health 1997 The new NHS: modern, dependable. The Stationery Office, London
Department of Health 1998 A first class service: quality in the new NHS. The Stationery Office, London
MMI Companies 1998 Transforming insights into clinical practice improvements: a 12-year data summary resource. MMI Companies, Deerfield, Illinois, USA
NATN 1994 Quality assessment document (QuAD). National Association of Theatre Nurses, Harrogate
NATN 1996 Risk assessment guide. National Association of Theatre Nurses, Harrogate
NATN 1998a Principles of safe practice in the perioperative environment. National Association of Theatre Nurses, Harrogate

NATN 1998b Safeguards for invasive procedures. National Association of Theatre Nurses, Harrogate

UKCC 1992 The code of professional conduct, 3rd edn. United Kingdom Central Council, London

Walshe K 1998 Cutting to the heart of quality. Health Management May: 20–21

Wilson J H 1992 Multidisciplinary pathways of care. Northern Regional Health Authority, Newcastle

Wilson J H 1996 Integrated care management: the path to success? Butterworth Heinemann, Oxford

Wilson J H 1998a The clinical negligence scheme for Trusts. British Journal of Nursing 6(20): 1166–1167

Wilson J H 1998b Incident reporting. British Journal of Nursing 7(11): 670–671

Accountability and the law in perioperative care

Martin Hind

All perioperative practitioners, in whatever setting they work, are accountable for their practice. This chapter examines key aspects of accountability of which perioperative practitioners should be aware, in their pursuit of high-quality and effective patient care.

RESPONSIBILITY AND ACCOUNTABILITY

It is important that perioperative practitioners understand the difference between responsibility and accountability since the terms are sometimes used interchangeably, which can lead to confusion. It would be useful to consider the work of Bergman (1981) who defines accountability from a set of preconditions. These are **ability**, **responsibility** and **authority**.

Ability relates to the knowledge, skills and values which underpin the role of perioperative practitioners in whatever setting they work. Perioperative care takes place in many different settings, with various types of surgical and anaesthetic techniques being employed. These areas of practice require specialist knowledge and skills in order to enable effective practice and there is little doubt that perioperative practitioners require ability to fulfil this role.

Responsibility refers to the tasks, roles and duties that are assigned to practitioners during their work within the perioperative environment. It links closely with the ability to practise, in that practitioners have many responsibilities within their role in whatever setting they work.

Authority refers to the freedom to make and act on decisions in the exercise of the professional role. The standard of patient care throughout the entire perioperative period relies heavily on the decisions and actions of practitioners.

Ability, responsibility and authority are inherent to these activities and there is little doubt that perioperative practitioners fulfil all these preconditions to being accountable, rather than merely responsible for their practice.

It may be easy to define accountability in this way but clarifying how perioperative practitioners may be held to account for their practice is more complex. This clarification is best achieved by considering the four ways in which accountability may be exercised.

1. Self
2. Legal

3. Contractual
4. Professional

SELF ACCOUNTABILITY

The self mode of accountability is the moral dimension that cannot be externally enforced on the individual. It is that sense of right or wrong that people instinctively possess. In the context of perioperative practice, if practitioners have knowledge, skills and experience then they are perfectly capable of knowing what is right and wrong in their practice. Marks-Maran (1993) has argued that this mode of accountability is the clarification of personal values in that there can be no prescriptions, laws, codes or job descriptions for moral accountability.

LEGAL ACCOUNTABILITY

The legal mode of accountability can be divided into criminal and civil law. Perioperative practitioners are accountable to the public through criminal law and accountable to the patient through civil law.

Fortunately, criminal charges in relation to care in any health-care arena are rare but it does sometimes happen. In the past, there have been cases where health-care professionals have been convicted of criminal offences committed while they were practising. Being engaged in professional practice does not exempt an individual from their responsibilities to society through criminal law. Peysner (1998) has suggested that nurses are most likely to risk prosecution for a criminal offence in areas where invasive procedures or physical examinations are performed without the consent of the patient. This may lead to prosecution for the crime of battery or under the Offences against the Person Act 1861. Issues relating to consent within the perioperative period will be considered later in this chapter.

Negligence

Civil actions occur when a patient sues under the law of negligence. This is sometimes referred to as litigation and the costs of this in the UK are rising every year. In 1995 the cost of negligence was £125 million, rising to £175 million in 1996 and £200 million in 1997. This figure is expected to continually rise and consume money that would otherwise be spent on patient care. One reason for this trend is that patients are becoming increasingly aware of their rights through initiatives such as the Patient's Charter and through the media.

It is well known that the operating department is an area of high risk and all practitioners need to be constantly aware of the possibilities of litigation. Missing swabs or instruments, diathermy burns, tissue or nerve damage due to incorrect positioning, drug errors, mix-ups with patients, wrong operations and invalid patient consent are just a few of the common risks. In addition to this, increasing pressures on available resources, recruitment and retention problems, communication breakdowns and conflicts among staff are all factors that may influence the occurrence of these risks. All perioperative practitioners have a key role to play in minimising these risks and ensuring that patients get the best and safest care and understanding how the law of negligence works is a useful way to achieve this.

Negligence is best defined as a failure in the duty of care owed to another with resultant harm to that person. Perioperative practitioners need to be aware of three key areas:

1. Duty of care
2. Standard of care
3. Causation

Duty of care

The legal test for the duty of care was established some time ago in a case entirely unrelated to health care, where a person drank a bottle of ginger beer and discovered a badly decomposed snail in the bottle (*Donoghue v Stevenson 1932* AC 562). It was found that the manufacturer of the drink owed a duty of care to the person who ultimately drank it. This case determined that a person must take 'reasonable care to avoid acts or omissions which she or he can reasonably foresee would be likely to injure a person directly affected by those acts'. This means that a duty of care exists between a practitioner and those people who could be affected by their actions or omissions. It follows, then, that a duty of care exists between practitioners and patients under their care. In fact, it is argued that there cannot be a closer legal relationship than that which exists between patients and their carers (Fulbrook 1995).

Standard of care

Once a duty of care is established, the next consideration is the standard of the care given and this is best explained by considering the Bolam test. The Bolam test arises from a case in which it was argued that the hospital was vicariously liable for the carelessness of a doctor who gave electroconvulsive therapy to a patient called Bolam without administering a relaxant drug or restraining the convulsive movements (*Bolam v Friern Barnet HMC 1957*). However, the court sought the opinion of other doctors who worked in this area of practice and they supported the actions of the doctor and Bolam lost the case.

The key point that arose from the Bolam case was not the clinical situation but the idea that the standard of care should be measured by other professionals who normally undertake the the same duties as the defendant. In the words of the judge: 'A doctor is not guilty of negligence if he has acted in accordance with a practice accepted as proper by a responsible body of medical men skilled in that particular art'. Since the early 1980s the Bolam test has been used in many cases and it is accepted that this test is now applied to all health-care professionals.

It was also established during the Bolam case that the standard would be that of the 'reasonably skilled and experienced professional'. This is a key point as it does not mean that practice has to be the best but that reasonable care has to be demonstrated which is supported by practitioners who are experienced in the relevant field of practice. The actions of the practitioner therefore need to be within the range of acceptable practice.

The standard of care expected of learners is also an important area to address as it is inappropriate to apologise to patients about mistakes being made simply because a learner made the mistake. The standard of care of learners was addressed in *Wilsher v Essex Area Health Authority* in 1986 (Case study 7.1).

Case study 7.1 Wilsher

Wilsher was a premature baby who had a number of clinical problems, including oxygen deficiency. His prospects of survival were poor and he was placed in a special care baby unit. During this time an inexperienced doctor was monitoring the baby's oxygen levels and mistakenly inserted a catheter into a vein rather than an artery. The doctor asked the senior registrar to check his work and the registrar failed to spot the mistake and some hours later, when replacing the catheter, made the same mistake himself. In both instances, the catheter monitor failed to register correctly the amount of oxygen in the baby's blood and the baby was given too much oxygen. The baby sustained retinal damage.

The junior doctor was not found to be negligent but only because he had asked for his work to be checked. Otherwise, he would clearly have been found negligent. The senior registrar was found to be negligent.
Wilsher v Essex Area Health Authority 1986 All ER 801

This case determined a key point about the standard of care regarding learners as it means that inexperience is no defence to an action for negligence. The law requires the trainee or learner to be judged by the same standard as their more experienced colleagues. Although the Wilsher case centred on the actions of doctors, the same principle applies to other health-care professionals and that would include perioperative practitioners and all learners in the perioperative environment.

Whoever is responsible for the supervision of learners must ensure that the standard of care which patients ultimately receive is maintained at an acceptable level. Conversely, learners should engage in the supervision process themselves by asking for their work to be checked. Supervision should be seen as a two-way process. This would also be true of practitioners working in new and unfamiliar areas of practice; there are responsibilities both ways to ensure that the standard of care is not breached. There need to be appropriate arrangements for the supervision of trainees and learners in the perioperative environment which, on the one hand, allow these learners to get experience while, on the other hand, protect the standard of care.

It can be very difficult to define how perioperative practitioners may be accountable when they often work under the direct supervision of surgeons and anaesthetists. Montgomery (1997) clarifies this point very well and explains that in a number of cases the courts have acknowledged the fact that health-care professionals work in teams, in which they have different responsibilities. The idea that each team member is expected to deliver the high standards of care that the team as a whole could offer has been rejected. The courts have also rejected the approach known as the 'captain of the ship' doctrine whereby professionals in charge of teams are responsible for the negligence of their members, even though they may not be personally at fault.

If, for example, a swab is left inside a patient during surgery the law recognises that it was the surgeon's responsibility to have checked that no swab was left inside rather than to be personally responsible for the scrubbed assistant's error. While the scrubbed assistant may be held liable for the error, the surgeon would be liable for failing to check. The same would apply in the case of the anaesthetic assistant. If the assistant draws up an incorrect anaesthetic dose, this does not make the anaesthetist negligent merely because he bore overall responsibility for anaesthesia (Montgomery 1997). The key point here is that professionals are responsible for their own mistakes and not for those of the members of their team.

However, the courts do recognise that a practitioner who relies on the instructions of the surgeon or anaesthetist is not negligent, even if these instructions turn out to be wrong at a later date. In other words, a practitioner who carries out an instruction given to them by the doctor which in hindsight may have been wrong will not be negligent if it was not obvious that the instruction was wrong. But practitioners are expected to challenge decisions on either procedural or substantive grounds if it appears, or it is blatantly obvious, that the instructions are wrong. It is no defence for the practitioner to state that they were merely following orders.

Causation

Causation has more to do with legal technicalities rather than being of great relevance to perioperative practitioners in their work. But it is possible for negligence to be established and the patient to eventually lose their case on the issue of causation. This happened in the Wilshire case where the baby was given too much oxygen and sustained retinal damage. While negligence on the part of the registrar was established, it was also found that the baby had an existing condition that could equally have caused the retinal damage. Because it was not clear whether the registrar's negligence or the pre-existing condition had caused the retinal damage, the case was lost.

Vicarious liability

Under the doctrine of vicarious liability the employers would be pursued by the patient's lawyers, simply because they would be more likely to be able to pay any compensation awarded in a successful action. But if the patient was harmed due to the negligence of an individual practitioner, or if they at least played a key role in the mistakes that led up to the incident, then in theory the practitioner could be pursued by the patient's lawyers. To date, there is no record of this having happened.

Issues to do with vicarious liability raise questions about new and developing roles in the perioperative environment. It is essential that practitioners are fully aware of the boundaries to their practice and that these are clarified and agreed with their employers. Vicarious liability operates on the basis that the practitioner was engaged in the duties that they were employed to undertake. There are many expanded and developing roles within the perioperative environment, including the surgeon's first assistant, surgeon's assistant, pre-assessment practitioner and many varied nurse practitioner roles. Both employers and practitioners need to be quite clear on the nature and purpose of these roles and the boundaries that are drawn up around them.

CONTRACTUAL ACCOUNTABILITY

The contractual mode of accountability involves the relationship between the practitioner and their employer, where there is a clear legal duty for employees to carry out the 'reasonable' orders of their employers.

Practitioners are responsible for fulfilling their contractual obligations as laid down in their job description within the guidance of the policies, procedures and standards that employers set. These guidelines all serve as parameters to the role and understanding these parameters is essential if practitioners are going to be in a position to properly account for their actions to their employers. If the practitioner fails to fulfil the reasonable expectations of their employers then the employers can take action against the practitioner.

Perioperative practitioners are often highly specialised and working in narrow fields of practice. It would be reasonable for the employer to provide appropriate training and support for a new role or for work in a different area which requires the utilisation of new knowledge and skills.

PROFESSIONAL ACCOUNTABILITY

The main reason for having this mode of accountability is to protect the patient. The principal function of a professional body is to maintain a register of qualified practitioners and to remove those who are unfit to practise because of a health problem or improper conduct. The professional body also normally oversees education and training matters but perhaps its primary function should be to regulate membership of the profession. This will normally be undertaken in a quasi-judicial process where a code of conduct provides the guiding principles by which practitioners are judged and therefore held accountable.

Nurses are professionally accountable to the United Kingdom Central Council for Nursing, Midwifery and Health Visiting (UKCC) in accordance with the principles set out in the *Code of professional conduct* (UKCC 1992). The UKCC accepts that professional accountability is concerned with weighing up the interests of patients in complex clinical situations (UKCC 1996). Practices within the perioperative arena reflect these complexities, where practitioners must use professional knowledge, judgement and skills to make decisions about patient care. Whatever actions are taken, or not as the case may be, the nurse must always be able to justify them. It should also be borne in mind that the UKCC advocates individual accountability in the same way that the law of negligence does.

Being accountable to a professional body is not an easy option. It is arguably the toughest of the external modes of accountability. It is tougher than the law and tougher than the practitioner's contractual obligations. This point is best explained by considering the similarities and differences between the different modes of accountability.

Although the different modes of accountability can be seen to converge within given practice situations, the key to understanding accountability is to grasp the fact that these modes work in different ways. While there may be similarities in the way they operate, there may also be different outcomes within each mode because each may be concerned with different aspects of the situation and may also have different standards of proof. This could be illustrated by making a general non-specific comparison between the legal and professional modes.

Tingle (1994) has observed that the law of negligence does not necessarily expect the professional to act as the patient's advocate, whereas a central plank of any form of professional accountability must be the imperative that members act as the patient's advocate in all aspects of their work. It can be seen, then, that patient advocacy is a critical concept within the professional mode of accountability.

A key difference, then, between the legal and professional modes of accountability is that the law of negligence is concerned with setting the minimum standard of care whereas the professional mode is concerned with promoting the highest standards of care (Montgomery 1997). A situation might arise where a practitioner acts within legal boundaries yet at the same time is in breach of their code of professional conduct.

INFORMED CONSENT

Informed consent has both legal and ethical dimensions; the ethical dimensions, in particular the principle of respect for autonomy, are covered in Chapter 8.

However, all perioperative practitioners need to be aware of the legal aspects of informed consent. It is a requirement of the law that competent adults provide their consent before they are touched during the course of any care and treatment they may receive. If a patient is touched and consent is not sought then the professional would have committed the crime of battery and the civil wrong of trespass to the person. It would be rare for such a situation to occur in the perioperative period, except perhaps if there was a major breakdown in communication and the patient received the wrong surgery. What is more likely is a situation whereby the process of seeking consent was faulty or improper. Problems with the level of disclosure, understanding on the part of the patient, the presence of coercion or undue influence or questions about the patient's competence could result in the patient suing under the law of negligence for a breach of the duty of care to inform the patient.

The principles of informed consent are enshrined in the Patient's Charter which tells patients that they have the right to have any proposed treatment, including any risks involved in that treatment and any alternatives, clearly explained to them before they decide whether to agree to it (DoH 1995).

Beauchamp & Childress (1989) identify five elements to consent.

1. Disclosure
2. Understanding
3. Voluntariness
4. Competence
5. Consent

These elements serve as a useful framework to consider the importance of the consent process throughout the perioperative period.

Disclosure

Patients undergoing surgery need to be given details about the procedure along with its expected outcomes and associated risks. The level of disclosure is best explained by returning to the concept of standard of care within the law of negligence (see Case study 7.2).

Case study 7.2   The Sidaway case

Sidaway had suffered from persistent neck and shoulder pain and was advised that she would need surgery to her spinal column to relieve the pain. The surgeon warned her of the possibility of disturbing the nerve root but did not warn her of the possibility of damage to the spinal cord itself even though the surgery would be within 3 mm of it. Sidaway consented to the operation, which was undertaken with due skill and care. During the operation the spinal cord was damaged and this resulted in Sidaway becoming severely disabled.

Sidaway sued the surgeon and the hospital governors, alleging that the surgeon had been in breach of his duty of care to inform her of the risks. Under the application of the Bolam test, Sidaway lost her case at the trial court, the court of appeal and the House of Lords.

Sidaway v Bethlem RHG 1985 1 All ER 643

The Sidaway case demonstrates that it is the Bolam test that determines the level of disclosure within the consent process.

Disclosure of information should not be seen as relating only to the surgery and anaesthesia but would also include all other care that the patient may receive throughout the perioperative period. Perioperative practitioners have a lead role in ensuring that adequate disclosure takes place throughout this entire process.

Understanding

Disclosure of information is not enough if the patient fails to understand it. Practitioners need to ensure that their patients understand fully the information given to them about all aspects of their care and treatment throughout the perioperative period. This might include clarifying information given by the doctor, in particular the proposed surgery. Concerns have been raised about the standard and quality of the 'consent for surgery' process, in particular where junior doctors are involved (Richardson et al 1996). Perioperative practitioners can play a key part in ensuring that the patient's understanding of their surgery, as well as other aspects of care, is maintained at a satisfactory level.

Voluntariness

This relates to the conditions under which consent may be sought. Patients who require surgery are vulnerable to the suggestion of well-meaning health-care professionals who may be clear about what needs to be done. It may be difficult to prevent some degree of coercion in securing consent from a patient but misrepresentation of the facts or overt manipulation of the patient should never occur.

Competence

Consent can only be valid if the patient is competent to give it. Some patients may not be legally or mentally competent to give consent and this is a complex area that cannot be fully explained within this chapter. However, in the perioperative environment there are a number of specific issues relating to competence that may arise, which do need consideration.

It may not be possible to seek the consent of a patient who is admitted unconscious and in need of life-saving surgery. In these circumstances, the professionals would clearly have a duty to act in the patient's best interests and for the surgery to go ahead, but only if it could be demonstrated that the situation was indeed life threatening. The same considerations would apply in a situation where, during an elective operation, the surgeon identifies the need for additional surgery unrelated to that which was consented for. If the new problem identified was life threatening then the surgeon may be justified in performing this additional procedure. However, if it is not a life-threatening problem then, under the law of trespass, it would be wrong for this additional procedure to be performed. The patient would need to be woken up and consulted properly under the usual consent process before this additional procedure could be performed.

Seeking consent from patients in the anaesthetic room may also be problematical, in particular when the patient is under the influence of a 'mind-altering' premedication. It would be very difficult, if not impossible, to demonstrate that all the requirements of a valid consent process had been met in these circumstances. It would therefore be wrong to seek consent from patients under these conditions.

Consent

Consent may be either 'implied' or 'expressed' and both methods can be found within the perioperative period. Implied consent occurs where patients indicate through action that they are willing for a particular act of care to take place, for example holding the arm out for a blood test or blood pressure measurement.

Expressed consent can be given either verbally or in writing. Written consent is vastly superior as evidence to all other methods of consent giving as it is a permanent record of the consent process. This is of particular use should a case arise at a later date in a court of law.

It is possible that a patient may be anaesthetised and on the operating table when it is discovered that there is no consent form signed but medical and ward staff are sure that the patient has consented to the planned surgery. Under normal practices this should not occur, as checking the consent form is a requirement of the preoperative preparation process. However, it is possible that the consent is still valid as verbal and implied consent are equally valid in law (Dimond 1990). This might indicate that the procedure could be performed. However, Dimond (1990) believes that it would be wiser to ensure that the patient had signed a consent form, meaning that the patient should be returned to the ward. It is stressed, though, that this situation should really be avoided in the first place with proper and effective consent-checking procedures during the preoperative period.

RECORD KEEPING

All records made within the perioperative period are potentially legal documents in that they could be used in complaints, investigations, professional conduct inquiries, coroner's courts and civil lawsuits. In particular, with ever-increasing litigation it is of even more importance that perioperative records reflect the highest standards of care. Ensuring that accurate and comprehensive perioperative records are kept is a key aspect of practitioners exercising accountability.

Records are 'any permanent form of information recorded about a patient or client' (Young 1995, p.179). These records may include perioperative care plans, records of care during surgery, drug charts, observation charts, accident/incident forms and transfer records. A number of key principles need to be considered when keeping perioperative records.

Contemporary

Perioperative records need to be completed as near as possible to the time of the events that they refer to. It may not always be possible to complete records during the process of giving care or responding to incidents but practitioners must ensure that they complete them in reasonable time after the event/incident.

Comprehensive

Perioperative records should be factual and informative about the events/incidents and should detail the responses and patient's progress. They should serve to clarify the care that was given and not be difficult to understand. For example, 'I took his BP, resps and sats and these were okay' is unclear and lacks sufficient detail to clarify to a lay person or solicitor what exactly happened. As a general rule, perioperative records should be written in such a way that patients themselves could understand them.

Legible and permanent

Perioperative records should be legible and abbreviations only used if they are commonly recognised and well known. Where mistakes in recording have been made, these should not be deleted but a line should be put through them to identify the mistake while also ensuring that it can be read at a later date should the need arise.

Perioperative records must always be written in permanent form; pencil should never be used and blue pen is not advisable because of poor photocopying properties.

Effective perioperative record keeping promotes best-quality patient care and safeguards the professional from legal or disciplinary action. It is essential that all perioperative practitioners adhere to effective record-keeping practices.

CONCLUSION

Perioperative practitioners are accountable for their practice in a number of ways. Grasping the complexities of this accountability is essential if high standards of patient care are to be maintained. There may well be tensions associated with the different modes of accountability and it is sometimes not easy for practitioners to know how to act or behave in certain circumstances. But the overriding rule is that the patients' interests must come before any conflicting personal or contractual interest.

Being accountable lies at the heart of the best of professional practice and this should remain the priority for all perioperative practitioners whatever role they play.

REFERENCES

Beauchamp T, Childress J 1989 Principles of biomedical ethics, 3rd edn. Oxford University Press, Oxford

Bergman J 1981 Accountability – definition and dimensions. International Nursing Review 28(2): 53–59

Department of Health 1995 The patient's charter and you. NHS Executive, Leeds

Dimond B 1990 Legal aspects of nursing. Prentice Hall, Hemel Hempstead

Fulbrook S 1995 Duty of care – (1). British Journal of Theatre Nursing 5(5): 18–19

Marks-Maran D 1993 Accountability. In: Tschudin V (ed) Ethics, nurses and patients. Scutari Press, Harrow

Montgomery J 1997 Health care law. Oxford University Press, Oxford

Peysner J 1998 Litigation. In: McHale J, Tingle J, Peysner J (eds) Law and nursing. Butterworth Heinemann, Oxford

Richardson N, Jones P, Thomas M 1996 Should house officers obtain consent for operation and anaesthesia? Health Trends 28(2): 56–59

Tingle J 1994 Perspectives on clinical negligence in the operating theatre. British Journal of Theatre Nursing 4(8): 7–8

UKCC 1992 Code of professional conduct, 3rd edn. United Kingdom Central Council, London

UKCC 1996 Guidelines for professional practice. United Kingdom Central Council, London

Young A 1995 Record keeping. British Journal of Nursing 4(3): 179

Ethical issues in perioperative care

Andy Mardell   Charles Laugharne

8

INTRODUCTION

We are called upon to make ethical decisions on a daily basis, both in our home life and at work. Essentially, ethics are issues of whether something is right or wrong or whether things are good or bad. Ethics are usually concerned with either the actions of individuals or the consequences of those actions. Within society, our ethical values are based upon social norms passed on to us through our family and other members of society. Religious beliefs and the law may also play an important part in developing our ethical values. People also adopt personal ethical values based on their own experience and knowledge.

Increasingly, professional groups, such as the United Kingdom Central Council for Nursing, Midwifery and Health Visiting (UKCC), have intervened in helping nurses to develop a professional ethic. Within perioperative care, nurses follow the *Code of professional conduct* as laid down by the UKCC (1992) while other professional groups may follow their own profession's codes. Whilst derived from similar ethical theories and principles, the emphasis on those theories may be different. For example, the degree to which you can harm an individual may vary between not at all, on one hand, to when it is justified by greater good, on the other. The situation is therefore rather pluralistic.

Additionally, ethics, rather than being clearcut, are most often associated with clarifying questions rather than finding absolute solutions. Although we are taught from an early age that we should not 'harm' other individuals, there are many legitimate and reasonable exceptions to this principle.

THEORIES OF ETHICS

Ethics, in a more formal academic sense, are part of moral philosophy. Philosophers as diverse as Aristotle, David Hume, Jeremy Bentham and Ivan Illich have developed useful theories with which to decide ethical questions. Although many people may be unaware of the works of these theorists, many of their ideas form the basis on which we regularly decide ethical issues. The major differences in ethical theories developed by these philosophers are largely based on their focus on a sequential process. Each principle is concerned with one aspect of that process, the process being, first, the characteristics of the individuals or their virtues, then people's actions and finally, the consequences of people's actions.

The first philosophical debates about ethics were undertaken in ancient Greece in around 350 BC. Aristotle and Socrates thought that people had inherent virtues that informed their ethical decision making. They thought that goodness was essentially that which is most appropriate to the task (Burnard & Chapman 1993). One could argue whether or not individuals are born with inherent virtues or if goodness could be defined by that which is most appropriate. To an extent, people can develop virtuous behaviour and also goodness may relate to intentions rather than appropriateness.

To an extent, this ethical theory has been applied to modern nursing. Florence Nightingale (1820–1910), for example, was of the belief that nurses should have inherent virtues such as honesty, sobriety and loyalty. The connection between nursing and religious orders would reinforce the connection between virtue and nursing practice. These virtues have been supported by writers such as Schrock (1980), Tschudin (1986) and even the UKCC (1992). Tschudin wrote that nursing ethics was based on an ethic of caring.

Deontology is an ethical theory very much applied in nursing practice. Developed by the German philosopher Immanuel Kant (1724–1804), this theory works on the principles of beneficence and non-maleficence. Beneficence is linked to the idea that we should always do good whereas non-maleficence means not doing harm. In health care, there are few situations where there are no likely risks of harm and the emphasis is usually on doing good, that is, beneficence. Kant believed that ethics came from duty and intent. What you do should not be based on consequences, over which we have little control, but on duty and an intention to do good. All we can do, therefore, is to look at the intentions of what people do; for example, the good intentions of a nurse delivering care without the consent of an unconscious victim of a road traffic accident.

Utilitarianism is perhaps the most widely know ethical theory. Developed in England by the philosophers Jeremy Bentham (1748–1832) and John Stuart Mill (1806–73), it is characterised by the slogan 'the greatest good for the greatest number'. Utilitarianism, in contrast to deontology, is based on the consequences of people's actions rather than their motives and intentions. It does not look at the process by which people come to an ethical decision but at what the outcomes of that decision would be. Many medical decisions are supported by this theory. Decisions as to which of four people will get the one kidney transplantation are based on outcomes and the greatest good. Also, leaving a 'dirty' or infected case till the end of the operating theatre list would be based on the greatest good. Generally, however, nurses cannot justify 'harm' of individuals on any basis of greater good. The *Code of professional conduct* states: 'Ensure that no action or omission on your part, or within your sphere of responsibility, is detrimental to the interests, condition or safety of patients and clients' (UKCC 1992).

There may therefore be some conflict here between medical ethics and nursing ethics.

PRINCIPLES

At a level below ethical theories are ethical principles which are somewhat easier to apply in practice. One set of principles mentioned in many nursing textbooks are those of autonomy, beneficence, non-maleficence and justice (Beauchamp & Childress 1994).

Autonomy is related to the subject's freedom. In reality, this is closely linked to informed consent; that there is enough information and that is comprehensible, with any decision being made freely by the subject. It also relates to confidentiality and the protection of individuals from the disclosure of private or harmful information. Beneficence is concerned with doing good whereas non-maleficence is not doing harm.

Finally, justice is about an individual's right to fair treatment. This could relate to the compromising of care; taking advantage of vulnerable groups by using them as subjects for research; or the ignoring of people's rights. These principles will often relate to laws and conventions and work on a global, regional or national level. Interestingly, Hebert (1996) sees the principles of autonomy, beneficence, non-maleficence and justice being removed in medicine because of the nature of medicine and the potential for harm in research.

Ethics questions present difficulties for all health professionals including nurses. There are several areas where ethics would play an important role in the decision making of perioperative care.

CONFIDENTIALITY

Perioperative nurses often have access to sensitive information concerning an individual in their care. Examples include women who are pregnant and will be undergoing a termination, people who have cancer or individuals who have an infectious disease such as AIDS. As in any other area of nursing, perioperative nurses have a duty to protect or safeguard information about an individual. This information should not be divulged, without permission, to any individual who does not have a right to that information.

The principle of confidentiality is derived from a number of sources. It is part of the system of common law, it is enshrined in ethical principles and codes including nursing's *Code of professional conduct* (UKCC 1992). There is always the danger that because of the familiarity of the situation, nurses may trivialise the information that they have access to and there is then a danger of a breach of confidentiality. Maintaining confidentiality is an important ethical principle and, in a practical sense, is essential if you wish people to share sensitive information with you. This is part of the nurses' role and is therefore important in allowing nurses to function in their work. There is also quite a diversity of situations where nurses must divulge information about an individual where there is no right to confidentiality. These would include a legal duty under a variety of acts: for example, if a criminal offence has been committed; where the disclosure is in the public interest; or where the person, acting in an official capacity, places information in the public domain.

Nevertheless, there are specific ethical issues in perioperative care. One of the most important breaches of confidentiality is in the distribution of theatre lists. One would have to question to what extent an operating list should be distributed and whether this should be displayed in an area with unrestricted access. It is relatively common to find lists that include the individual's name, address and operation displayed at the nurses' station on a surgical ward. The list may also include information about the likely infection risk of the individual or whether the patient has cancer. Often a list is photocopied complete and distributed widely to individuals who only have an interest in certain aspects of the information.

ADVOCACY

Many nurses feel that they act as advocates for their patients by acting in their best interests. The concept is enshrined in the UKCC *Code of professional conduct* that states that nurses should: 'act always in such a manner so as to promote and safeguard the interests and well being of patients and clients' (UKCC 1992).

The *Concise Oxford Dictionary* defines an advocate as 'one who pleads or speaks for another' and according to Burnard & Chapman (1993) this is a misunderstood concept. Advocacy of the types mentioned above are not controversial as they enshrine values with which nurses will agree. There will undoubtedly be many occasions when nurses are required to use their skills of empathy and their frequent personal interaction with a patient to mediate between the patient and other health-care professionals (Burnard & Chapman 1993). This will be particularly true when patients are unable to speak for themselves or when a person is weak or vulnerable. Patients will turn to nurses to advise them, to interpret information they have received or to give guidance about treatment or care and what other alternatives may exist that the patient and their family may consider.

One view of advocacy in nursing comes from the philosophical perspective. Gadow (1983) describes a concept called 'existential advocacy' which suggests that individuals be assisted by nursing to *authentically* (original italics) exercise their freedom of self-determination. 'Authentic' is defined as being a way of reaching decisions that are truly one's own, decisions that express all that one believes about oneself and the world, the entire complexity of one's values.

Ellis (1992) develops the notion by viewing the actions of the advocate from both a consequentialist and non-consequentialist perspective. The consequentialist view is that decisions should be made to achieve the greatest all-round good. Ellis (1992) cites Murphey & Hunter (1984) who point out that:

> The professional, while being obliged to act in the patient's best interests, is not permitted to define that interest in any way contrary to the patient's definition: it is not the professional but the patient that shall define what 'best interests' shall mean.

Ellis maintains that the non-consequentialist view is that actions that are good in themselves should be implemented and that those which are wrong in themselves should be avoided.

Allmark & Klarzynsky (1992) attack the notion that nurses can or should act as patients' advocates. Whilst conceding that nurses may be in the position of pleading the case for a patient, they pose two questions.

1. To whom or against whom are nurses advocating?
2. What exactly should nurses be pleading?

It is suggested that the growth of advocacy is in part due to the growth of empowerment for patients, usually against doctors. Advocacy in nursing is, according to Allmark & Klarzynsky (1992), part of a political struggle for power between doctors and nurses and as such can be viewed as 'empire building'.

Kendrick (1994) suggests that there is tremendous disparity between the central players in the health-care equation. The all-powerful, all-knowing doctor is contrasted with the unselfish, caring nurse and the patient as helpless and utterly trusting. Kendrick suggests that if the power in this equation were equal then the need for advocacy would be greatly diminished, if not 'totally debunked'! This is supported by Adams, cited in Penn (1994), who states: 'The need for advocacy is the result of the failure of the healthcare structure to function as it should'.

Cahill (1994) gives the example of a doctor refusing to discuss a terminal illness with a patient who then turns to a nurse for information. In the role of the true advocate, the nurse would discuss with the doctor why the decision to withhold information was made and what evidence exists to support the contention that the outcome will be beneficial or that the act is right. Either response, to tell the truth or go along with the doctor, can, according to Cahill, be defended. In ignoring the request and withholding the truth, the nurse could claim not to be lying by appealing to principles of beneficence or non-maleficence, arguing that knowledge of the facts may be harmful to the patient. This would be supported on utilitarian grounds but not on deontological grounds as many deontologists believe that deception is wrong for reasons independent of its consequences.

If, then, the position of the nurse advocate is difficult in general, what are the implications for perioperative nurses who wish to advocate for their patients? The fact that there is very little written about advocacy in the perioperative setting is recognition of the difficulty faced by nurses in this respect. Wiseman (1990) suggests that advocacy for the perioperative nurse exists on two levels: active and passive. In the passive mode, nurses support the patient as long as their needs are congruent with the needs of those in authority, so that the nurses' actions stem from their expectations and not their own beliefs. In the active role, nurses' actions originate from personal and professional beliefs that stem from what is morally right on behalf of the patient.

It is worth considering whether perioperative nurses, faced with difficult ethical decisions in the theatre and often acting on behalf of unconscious patients, could ever truly act as an advocate in any sense. To do so would require an in-depth knowledge of all medical or surgical alternatives to any form of treatment, including side-effects and outcomes. A knowledge of alternative therapies and their success rates might also be useful. This is quite apart from an understanding of what the patient would want if they were conscious or able to make an informed decision for themselves. This would require visiting the patient preoperatively, which many perioperative nurses do, and entering into a detailed discussion of the surgery and decisions that the patient has made. The discussion should cover all possible eventualities and courses of action that may occur. Consideration should also be given to whether all this information should be recorded somewhere and whether the surgeon who is to carry out the operation (assuming it is known who it will be) should be involved at this point. Armed with this information the perioperative nurse could then confidently guide the surgeon as to the wishes of the patient during the operation. In reality, it is more likely that the nurse will act in the role described by Wiseman (1990) as the passive advocate or even as the consequentialist as described by Ellis (1992), whereby decisions are taken to achieve the greatest all-round good and not to question the authority of the surgeon or management.

In the rush to embrace advocacy, it appears that nurses and practitioners in general have not taken stock of precisely what the term means. To some extent, this is not surprising as there is no clear agreement as to which definition of advocacy is appropriate in the context of nursing or health care. Yet without a fundamental understanding of this most elusive concept, it is doubtful whether health-care professionals can reasonably be expected to be advocates for their patients.

Advocacy, as described by some theorists, means providing patients or clients with any information they require and respecting any decisions they may make based on that information. From the legal perspective, the advocates would be required to act for the patient in supporting them in exercising their choice. Whether or not the nurse agrees with the decision is immaterial under either version of advocacy. In supporting the patient, the position of the practitioner as advocate is both unclear and untested in law.

The position of perioperative nurses as members of the health-care team also makes advocacy difficult. Whilst advocating for patients will not always bring them into a conflict situation, there is the potential for nurses to find themselves in a precarious position. In this role, nurses may ultimately be faced with the prospect of a disagreement with their employer as well as a member of the medical profession. The position of perioperative nurses is probably even more precarious as they work closely with medical staff and are less likely to know exactly what the patient would want under all given circumstances. The knowledge that the nurse possesses will be crucial in this scenario in stating the case for the patient/client and the practitioner. If their knowledge of advocacy, the law and the alternatives is found wanting then practitioners may find themselves facing disciplinary action or dismissal from their employment.

What is apparent is that the term 'advocacy' is being used to describe caring and doing the best thing for patients. This is something that nurses and other health-care professionals have always done and should continue to do.

INFORMED CONSENT

Informed consent is one of the most important considerations in perioperative nursing. Informed consent is two concepts rather than one single concept. First, it requires that sufficient information is given in order to make a decision and that the information can be comprehended by the individual. Second, that a decision is made wholly without any pressure to make a decision one way or the other. Informed consent is enforced in law and therefore is not simply a matter of ethical principles or values being honoured. Having said that, the perioperative nurse acts more like a checker of documentation rather than someone who is legally responsible for informed consent. This is usually because the nurse is not able to give the amount of detailed information that the patient needs to allow them to make a decision. The surgeon is therefore legally required to obtain informed consent. The patient may need, however, to understand the nurse's role in relation to perioperative care in order to give true informed consent. These explanations may be given at any time from admission to the point where the client or patient is taken to theatre. In reality, true informed consent is rarely obtained.

Ethical dilemmas with informed consent will usually arise where it is not possible to obtain informed consent for a surgical procedure or where the nurse suspects that the patient has not been given full information on the procedure that will be undertaken. The nurse will regularly come across patients who have limited knowledge of the procedure to which they have consented.

Nurses do have a professional responsibility to obtain informed consent for the interventions that they carry out. So, the nurse should first and foremost obtain permission to undertake any procedure on an individual; however, this is not always possible. In a similar way to nurses working in an intensive care unit, perioperative nurses often find themselves in a position where patients are not able to judge whether or not to undergo a nursing intervention. They may be unconscious or under the influence of neurologically acting drugs. Consent should be obtained well before the time of the intervention, if at all possible.

The second big area of concern today is in regard to the rights of children. A busy children's day surgery unit may see hundreds of children each week from a wide age range. The issue has become more important since the introduction of The Children Act (DoH 1989) and a number of cases regarding the rights of individuals under the age of 16 years. Generally, it is believed that consent for a child under 16 years should be obtained through a parent or guardian. It is recognised that a child as young as 12 years (or younger) may be in a position to give informed consent but in terms of good nursing practice, it seems wise to obtain consent from both the child and the parents. The degree of control that an individual has over what happens to them has been shown to have a positive effect on outcomes. Nurses would therefore, purely on the basis of health outcomes, wish to obtain consent of even a child to a procedure.

There is also the ethical difficulty of obtaining informed consent from an adult for someone who is quite capable of giving consent themselves. The 'Gillick case' highlights the dilemma. In this case, a mother objected to her daughter, who was under the age of 16 years, being given contraceptive advice by her health authority without the mother's permission. The child was considered competent to give informed consent in this instance. The case went some way to defining how that competence may be determined. Richardson & Webber (1995) describe 'Gillick competence' as: 'to have sufficient maturity to understand the nature of the proposed treatment and the capacity to make a decision in their own right'. There is a need, therefore, for perioperative nurses to establish an understanding of development in childhood and support the increasing rights of children in their care.

CONSCIENTIOUS OBJECTION

Nurses are also cultural beings and therefore some of their beliefs may conflict with the work they do. The mechanism of protection of the values and beliefs is enshrined in the *Code of professional conduct*: 'Make known to an appropriate person or authority any conscientious objection which may be relevant to professional practice' (UKCC 1992).

There may be many issues that a nurse might consider morally wrong. Generally, nurses may find assisting with terminations against their moral beliefs and nurses can opt not to participate in these. However, an abortion may be essential for the survival of the mother and would nurses be ethically right to refuse to assist in this case? Would this be an act of unprofessional conduct? Several other procedures that nurses may find it difficult to assist with include neurosurgery for mental health clients, electroconvulsive therapy, multiple organ transplantation and research on human subjects during the perioperative period in which they may be assisting but have little knowledge of or influence over what is done.

CULTURAL ISSUES

It has been suggested that one source of ethical principles that inform our decision making is our culture. This will be embedded in our family life, our social life and in law. It also follows that different cultural groups may arrive at different ethical decisions in similar circumstances, based on different values about what is good and right. One has to recognise a broad definition of the term 'culture'. It can be applied not only to different races but also to different ethnic groups, social groups and religious groups. In fact, today, most people belong to a diverse collection of complex cultural groups.

Although it is rather a cliché to suggest that nurses should recognise the cultural values of an individual, the reality is often very difficult. Most codes of practice enshrine this belief. The International Council's *Code for nurses* (1973) states: 'The nurse, in providing care, respects the beliefs, values and customs of the individual'. The UKCC *Code of professional conduct* (1992) supports this view: 'Take account of the customs, values and spiritual beliefs of patients/clients'.

There are several problems with this philosophy. First, given the heterogeneity of cultures in society, perioperative nurses cannot be expected to be aware of an individual's cultural beliefs and values in anything but a superficial way. Second, some very difficult ethical decisions based on culture have had to be settled by the courts where there has been a conflict between the beliefs of a cultural group and the professional responsibilities of the health-care group. An example is the religious reasons why Jehovah's Witnesses decide not to transfuse blood to save lives and the ethical difficulties this presents to other individuals working from a different set of ethical principles.

DIGNITY

Dignity is an unalienable human right and as such is included in the UKCC *Code of professional conduct*: 'The nurse must recognise the uniqueness and dignity of each patient and client...' (UKCC 1992). This will present differing challenges to nurses wherever they practise and this applies equally in the setting of the operating theatre.

The dignity of the perioperative patient is particularly important when they are under a general anaesthetic. Most perioperative nurses will be familiar with the scenario of the naked patient left exposed on the operating table while the surgical team are 'scrubbing up', sometimes for 5 minutes or so. Under such circumstances the question arises whether dignity is being compromised as the patient is unaware of what is happening. Since it is unlikely that many people would choose to lie naked in a room full of strangers if they were conscious and in an unnatural and dependent situation, we could conclude that this situation is undignified (Thompson et al 1994). We might also consider how they might feel if ever they were to find out. We might conclude that by exposing a person in this way, we dehumanise ourselves as well as the patient. It is not only the action of exposure but the way that such an exposure is treated. It would demonstrate respect for the individual if we were not to remove coverings until the last possible moment.

Dignity may be related to an individual's perception of what they perceive as 'proper'. Perioperative nursing may in many ways reduce patient care down to an almost conveyer-belt quality. This is not necessarily just a characteristic of modern surgical procedures such as day surgery but also more conventional inpatient nursing care. For example, the preparation of patients for theatre is often impersonal; putting on standardised theatre attire prior to surgery to an extent devalues the experience to that of a routine factory production line. The standard check, starving, nil by mouth, the routine nature of bathing, premedication and the constant monitoring at various stages of the journey to the anaesthetic room may result in the patient's dignity as an individual being compromised.

The question of death with dignity is another area that perioperative nurses deal with on a regular basis. There can be few things more distressing than being left to deal with the body of a person who has had their organs removed. Since the person has already been certified as 'brain dead' before reaching the operating theatre, it is questionable whether in this case there can be any realistic expectation of death with dignity. Much of the discussion in this area would rest on defining what dignity is. The German philosopher Immanuel Kant defined dignity as 'an intrinsic, unconditioned, incomparable worth or worthiness' (1972). This sense of worth is an important issue in this area since it is unlikely that nurses in the perioperative setting would know what patients would have wanted for themselves in the situation. Johnston (1989) suggests that persons have intrinsic worth and thus ought to be treated as ends in themselves rather than as mere means to the ends of others.

THE ETHICAL ENVIRONMENT

It can be seen that an ethical environment is far from being clear and in fact is a complex multidimensional phenomenon. Despite the formulation of ethical theories, ethical principles and codes of practice, not all situations can be resolved easily where there is an ethical dilemma. Some principles may conflict or the interpretation of codes may be open to dispute. The solution is using a well worked out framework for ethical decision making. One suggestion by Tadd (1998) is a five-stage process. It involves being 'morally alert', clarifying 'details of the situation', determining 'possible alternative actions', evaluating 'alternative actions' and 'making a decision'. It could be argued that these stages are important considerations in any decision-making process and not just that related to ethical issues.

Being 'morally alert' means understanding the cultural values of others and recognising those issues that are likely to lead to ethical dilemmas. It is also necessary to be alert to the way that different players within health care place differing perspectives on those values and beliefs. Awareness of issues can be increased initially by opening a dialogue with others and by attempting to understand their values and beliefs. From an educational perspective, becoming alert to ethical issues will be increased by reflecting on practice within an ethical context and by adoption of a more questioning approach. An understanding of customs, the law and the rights of individuals, as well as ethics, will increase the knowledge nurses can apply to practice.

Having become aware of these issues, the process of considering the alternatives and their worth before deciding on the best course of action is lengthy. Perioperative care can often be led by the need for urgency or deadlines as patients move through the system. It is not always possible to consider ethical issues in depth since nurses may be forced to make decisions quickly. It is therefore important to recognise potential issues as soon as possible and the study of ethics needs to be considered as a key issue within perioperative care. Given the vulnerable position patients often find themselves in during this period, these issues can be extremely important.

The resolution of ethical dilemmas with patients undergoing surgery may not be given due consideration. With the need to reduce waiting lists and the emphasis on health gain, other factors can inhibit the clarification of issues and the consideration of alternatives. Within perioperative care, there are real difficulties with applying ethical theories, principles and professional codes but in this area, there would seem to be a real potential to raise awareness of ethical issues and safeguard the rights and beliefs of the individual.

REFERENCES

Allmark P, Klarzynsky R 1992 The case against nurse advocacy. British Journal of Nursing 2(1): 33–36

Beauchamp T L, Childress J F 1994 Principles of biomedical ethics, 4th edn. Oxford University Press, Oxford.

Burnard P, Chapman C 1993 Professional and ethical issues in nursing. Scutari Press, Harrow

Cahill J 1994 Are you prepared to be their advocate? Professional Nurse 9(6): 371–375

Department of Health 1989 The Children Act 1989: an introductory guide for the NHS. Department of Health, London

Ellis P 1992 Role of the nurse advocate. British Journal of Nursing 1(1): 40–43

Gadow S 1983 Existential advocacy: philosophical foundation of nursing. In: Murphy C, Hunter H (eds) Problems in the nurse–patient relationship. Allyn & Bacon, Boston

Hebert P 1996 Doing right: a practical guide to ethics for physicians and medical trainees. Oxford University Press, Oxford

International Council of Nurses 1973 Code for nurses; ethical concepts applied to nursing. ICN, Geneva

Johnston M 1989 Bio ethics. A nursing perspective. W B Saunders, Sydney

Kant I 1972 The moral law (trans. H J Paton). University Press, London

Kendrick K 1994 An advocate for whom – doctor or patient? Professional Nurse 9(12): 826–829

Penn K 1994 Patient advocacy in palliative care. British Journal of Nursing 3(1): 40–42

Richardson J, Webber I 1995 Ethical issues in child health care. Mosby, London

Schrock R 1980 A question of honesty in nursing practice. Journal of Advanced Nursing 5(2): 135–148

Tadd W 1998 Ethical issues in nursing and midwifery practice: a perspective from Europe. Macmillan, Basingstoke

Thompson I, Melia K, Boyd K 1994 Nursing ethics. Churchill Livingstone, Edinburgh

Tschudin V 1986 Ethics in nursing: the caring relationship. Heinemann, London

UKCC 1992 Code of professional conduct for the nurse, midwife and health visitor. United Kingdom Central Council, London

Wiseman S J 1990 Patient advocacy. AORN Journal 51(3): 754–762

Changing roles, changing titles in the perioperative environment

Jacqueline F M Younger

INTRODUCTION

The roles of operating department staff have changed considerably over the last 20 years. Nurses and operating department practitioners (ODPs) are now sharing some aspects of patient care and are carrying out some activities that were traditionally performed by doctors. The reasons for developing new roles and the key principles which employers and employees should consider need to be explored in detail. However, the developments within perioperative care cannot be looked at in isolation. It is necessary to look at the wider health service issues and how demands on health-care providers have led to many new role developments.

BACKGROUND

Since the late 1980s two key themes have developed in parallel and these have had a major impact on health-care delivery.

1. Great emphasis has been placed on the team approach within all patient care settings.
2. The need to reduce junior doctors' hours has led to non-medical personnel being trained to undertake some duties which were previously the preserve of doctors.

The team approach

The Bevan Report (1989), *The management and utilisation of operating departments*, observed that although ODPs are trained to fulfil many roles in the operating theatre, they are often employed solely to assist the anaesthetist. Similarly, nurses with both anaesthetic and surgical skills are often not using their anaesthetic training. More flexibility might be achieved if staff were able to move freely between anaesthetics, surgery and the recovery room. Enabling staff to become competent in all these areas depends on managers having a positive approach to multiskilling and teamwork. Staff need to be given the opportunity to utilise their existing skills while others may need time to refresh their skills or train in new areas. Operating department staff are in short supply and to prevent constant list cancellations, multiskilling and combined approaches to training operating room staff and flexible working are becoming commonplace.

Multiskilling can be described as having more than one practised ability. It should not be seen as creating a jack of all trades, nor as taking over the roles of others. It should be the enhancement of practice to become expert in more than one area.

As Bevan (1989) highlighted, multiskilling is an effective means of human resource management. But, for it to be effective, the establishment levels need to be appropriate to allow staff to cross over into new areas, working alongside others as they learn. Excess sickness absence which reduces staffing levels and prevents development must be actively addressed, clinical teaching staff need to be available to support the learning, courses need to be accessible for theoretical backing and practical skill acquisition must be facilitated.

Development of the role of the operating department support worker has become necessary as qualified staff take on more duties. Support workers are invaluable in carrying out tasks like transporting patients to and from theatre, assisting with cleaning and waste disposal, ordering supplies and stocking up, caring for equipment and assisting with sterile services. Previously, education for this group of staff has been provided by in-house programmes but as National Vocational Qualifications (NVQs) for support workers develop they should be accessed to ensure that national competencies are acquired. The National Association of Theatre Nurses (NATN) has produced helpful guidelines for employers entitled *The role of the support worker* (NATN 1996).

In 1992 the Department of Health commissioned Greenhalgh and Company to undertake research into the interface between junior doctors and ward nurses. It was expected that some activities traditionally carried out by junior doctors could be performed by appropriately trained nurses. That report, published in 1994, included a recommendation to promote team-based approaches to patient care and to encourage the sharing of some duties between nurses and doctors. Six activities were found to take up 11–16% of junior doctors' time on wards. These were taking patient histories, venous blood sampling, inserting peripheral cannulae, referring patients for investigation, writing discharge letters and administering intravenous drugs. There was no statistical evidence to show a difference in outcome if these tasks were carried out by nurses. Hence, if nurses could undertake these activities there might be a reduction in the demands made on junior doctors' time. It was recommended, however, that these activities become part of all qualified nurses' roles rather than creating specialists and that the experience of collaborative practice and the six activities should be included in the preregistration training of nurses and in the undergraduate training of doctors.

The UKCC published the *Scope of professional practice* in 1992 which encouraged nurses to enhance their practice as they saw fit and move away from certification for extended roles. This document still provides the basis for ensuring that nursing practice remains dynamic and is able to meet changing health-care needs. It also included clear statements about training for new roles and accountability.

The general theme in all these documents has been to place great emphasis on team work and the opportunities available for medical and non-medical staff to share certain aspects of patient care.

Reducing junior doctors' hours

In 1987, the UK Health Departments published the report *Achieving a balance* which set out proposals for future medical manpower planning. The principal need it outlined was an increase in the number of consultants to provide leadership for the profession and to create opportunities for the expansion of the service. It recommended that the number of doctors in training grades should match the future number of consultants required. It also recommended that the number of training-grade doctors should be adequate to support consultants.

In 1991, the NHS Management Executive published *The new deal*. This document sought to limit the number of hours worked by junior doctors. This has led to the appointment of non-medical professionals to undertake some tasks previously done by doctors or to existing non-medical staff enhancing their practice to share some aspects of patient care.

The Calman Report (1993), *Hospital doctors: training for the future*, was produced to bring UK medical training into line with Europe and hence reduce the number of years spent in training grades. This was to be achieved by the introduction of a unified training grade (the specialist registrar) and by increasing protected teaching time for junior hospital doctors. The net result of the 'Calmanisation' of medical training would be a reduction in the service commitment of doctors in training.

Then in 1995, the Audit Commission Report *The doctors' tale* attempted to provide an overview of medical practice. The report included a section on skill mix and the deployment of other professionals but emphasised that clear job descriptions and adequate training are required as professional roles change.

As new roles have developed for non-medical personnel, several studies have set out to explore the benefits or otherwise of these developments. The following summarises a few of note.

An evaluation of nurse practitioner pilot projects was undertaken in 1994 by South Thames Regional Health Authority and Touche Ross Management Consultants. An evaluation of 20 pilot sites was undertaken where nurse practitioner roles had been introduced in primary, hospital and community care settings. The key findings were that:

- the workload of those undertaking new roles was diverse and this was linked to parameters being set locally;
- patients were satisfied by the care given by practitioners;
- nurse practitioners provided a safe and valued service;

- nurse practitioners extended the style and content of services but did not wholly replace the medical staff within the clinical setting in which they were working.

Also in 1994, Read & Graves reported on the *Reduction of junior doctors' hours in Trent Region: the nursing contribution*. During 1993 the Trent Regional Task Force for Junior Doctors Hours pump-primed numerous new nursing posts which were created specifically to reduce the hours of junior doctors. The Sheffield Centre for Health and Related Research (SCHARR) was commissioned to assess the impact of those posts. A multiple case study approach was used with cross-case comparison being made where possible. Thirty two roles in 16 clinical settings were assessed to establish the effects on junior doctors' workload, improvements in the quality of patient care, training of post holders and policy and organisational issues. The report concluded that the nursing posts it assessed had already made an important impact on junior doctors' workload and would continue to do so as the post holders gained more confidence. Both consultants and junior doctors perceived that patient care had improved since the introduction of the roles and that these posts should be continued.

Recommendations included:

- sharing expertise between post holders;
- ensuring that new roles did not reduce junior doctors' training opportunities;
- ensuring multiprofessional collaboration when developing new roles;
- ensuring that the training needs of post holders are given particular attention;
- examining the salary grading for post holders;
- examining the legal framework and policy issues which may be relevant.

It was also recommended that the Department of Health address several issues related to advanced nursing practice including training, nurse prescribing, nurse consenting, nurses requesting investigations and nurse referrals.

Further work was also recommended and the NHS Executive funded extra time for the production of the report *Catching the tide* (Read 1995). Lessons learned by the participants in the earlier study were used to give practical advice about role development.

In 1995 the National Nursing, Midwifery and Health Visiting Advisory Committee of the Scottish Office Department of Health undertook to consider new roles within nursing in Scotland and the wider United Kingdom (Scottish Office Department of Health 1995a,b). The survey set out to explore the range and scope of role developments, educational and managerial issues, implications of role development for working practices, the benefits or otherwise, role evaluation and future plans. Eighteen NHS trusts in Scotland were visited and it was reported that:

- the UKCC's *Scope of professional practice* (1992), together with the implications of *The new deal* (NHS Management Executive 1991), had been major catalysts in the development of new roles;
- a variety of attitudinal rather than evaluative barriers to development were expressed. The need for education and support was recognised;
- benefits outweighed drawbacks;
- in some trusts, legal issues were of concern;
- the use of protocols and evaluation techniques was still being developed;
- evaluations suggested that nurses were motivated about the developments and that new roles were successful.

In 1997 a nationwide database was set up to share information on new role development. The *Exploring new roles in practice* (ENRiP) study (King's Fund 1997) was commissioned by the Department of Health and the first stage of the study was to undertake a mapping exercise of five trusts in each of the eight NHS regions. The database produced provides information on 838 roles with a plethora of titles, parameters and salary grades. Although it is not an all-inclusive database, it does provide a picture of innovation around the country and guidelines have been produced for people to build their own database.

The second phase of the study took an in-depth look at 30 of the roles identified in the original mapping exercise and the document *Developing new roles in practice: an evidence-based guide* (Levenson & Vaughan 1999) is now available.

Box 9.1 A database for your area may be available

Within the author's own area, the NHS Centre for Reviews and Dissemination has produced the Anglia and Oxford Database of Practice and Service Developments (1997). The database contains brief details of developments within the Anglia and Oxford Region as stated by respondents in a survey undertaken between March and June 1997.

NEW ROLES IN PERIOPERATIVE PRACTICE

The studies discussed so far have focused on role development within the broadest health-care settings. However, one document which focused on the development of roles for non-medical staff within perioperative care was compiled by the NATN (1997). This document, produced as guidance for organisations and employers, defined the roles within perioperative care and discussed the main principles which should be considered when developing new roles, many of which have been referred to in the earlier studies.

The particular roles which have developed within perioperative care are discussed in more detail now.

The first assistant

Clarification is needed between the USA definition of the registered nurse first assistant (RNFA) and that used in the UK. In the USA, the Association of Operating Room Nurses (AORN 1984) provided an official statement defining the role, stating that RNFAs carry out the functions necessary to assist the surgeon in performing a safe operation. They practise perioperative nursing and, having attended further training and instruction, possess the necessary skills to assist the surgeon under direct supervision. RNFAs do not act as scrub nurses whilst performing their first assistant duties.

RNFA duties may include tissue handling, providing exposure, using instruments, suturing and providing haemostasis. Preparation for the RNFA role includes an RNFA course and internship geared towards nurses who have already received their nursing diploma or degree and who have had 2 years' perioperative experience (Rothrock 1987).

The AORN and the American College of Surgeons (ACS) recognise that ideally the first assistant to the surgeon should be a qualified surgeon or surgical resident but attainment of this ideal is not realistic in many hospitals so it is acceptable to utilise appropriately trained non-medical personnel. These personnel are not authorised to operate independently.

Variations in patient population, environment and state nurse practice legislation will influence the degree to which the role develops and duties are undertaken. The RNFA may well undertake duties which would be within the role of a surgeon's assistant in the UK.

In the UK, the role of the nurse as first assistant in the operating department (NATN 1993) is defined as:

> The role undertaken to provide skilled assistance, under direct supervision of the Surgeon. At no time will the activities undertaken be described as surgical intervention. Duties undertaken by the first assistant may include:
>   Skin preparation
>   Draping
>   Assisting with haemostasis
>   Assisting with cutting sutures/ligatures
>   Retracting organs
>   Handling instruments and tissue
>   Performing skin closure (not other layers).

Nurses and ODPs have acted as first assistant for many years during surgical procedures, when medical staff have been unavailable. However, they increasingly find themselves in the difficult position where they are expected to act as first assistant and instrument nurse/practitioner. Obviously, working in this dual capacity may have associated risks, especially if staffing levels elsewhere in the operating room are depleted. The primary role of perioperative staff should not be compromised.

The dilemma of acting in the dual capacity of first assistant and scrubbed instrument nurse/practitioner (not allowed in the USA) also raises concern regarding legal and professional issues which need to be considered by individuals and employers.

Unlike RNFAs, operating department staff acting as first assistants in the UK are not required to undertake formal training. The English National Board (ENB) for Nursing, Midwifery and Health Visiting does provide the N77 course *The nurse as first surgical assistant* which may be provided as a module of a BSc(Hons) Nursing Practice programme. However, there is nothing that stipulates that operating department staff acting as first assistants must complete this course and it is doubtful that such a ruling will be implemented in the future.

The surgeon's assistant

In 1989, a pilot scheme in Oxford was undertaken to evaluate the role of the non-medical practitioner assisting with cardiac surgical procedures. The cardiac surgeon's assistant was to be trained to:

- actively assist with operations (including saphenous vein harvest);
- assess patients pre- and postoperatively;
- undertake wound-healing research;
- assist with the training of junior medical staff.

The pilot was approved by the Royal College of Surgeons (RCS) and the Department of Health (DoH) despite strong criticism from the medical profession. The person appointed was to train in the surgical skills required to remove saphenous veins by attending the physicians' assistant training programme at the Cleveland Clinic in Ohio, USA. The Oxford project was evaluated by the RCS and DoH in 1992 and since then the role of surgeon's assistant has developed throughout the UK in many specialities (see Box 9.2).

The role of the surgeon's assistant is: 'the role undertaken to provide skilled assistance *and* some surgical intervention under the supervision of a surgeon' (NATN 1994).

> *The duties of a surgical assistant may include:*
> *Assessing patients preoperatively*
> *Assisting the surgeon by carrying out some invasive*
> *   procedures (harvesting saphenous vein, cystoscopy, wound closure)*
> *Participating in postoperative care*
> *Undertaking evaluation of care.* (NATN 1997)

The potential benefits of the surgical assistant role include:

- reduction in cancellations due to the proactive preoperative assessment role;
- improvement in wound healing. As surgical assistants become competent they provide a consistent standard of wound closure and are available to teach junior doctors wound closure techniques;
- junior doctors have more time to shadow senior medical staff, attend training sessions and focus on essential medical duties.

Each speciality has set up the new roles in its own way to meet local needs so there is a lack of consistency. Concern has been expressed about the haphazard way in which the surgeon's assistant role has evolved.

Box 9.2 Examples of specialities in which surgical assistant roles have evolved	
Cardiac	Pre- and postoperative assessment of patients, harvesting saphenous vein and radial artery as vascular conduits and wound closure
Orthopaedics	Pre- and postoperative assessment of patients, assisting in theatre and wound closure
Endoscopy	Performing limited flexible endoscopy in coloproctology and gastroenterology and screening patients prior to referral for medical assessment
Laparoscopy	Pre- and postoperative assessment of patients, inserting ports and directly assisting with surgery
Urology	Assessing patients pre- and postoperatively, initiating primary investigations prior to referral for medical assessment and assisting in theatre
Gynaecology	Assessing patients preoperatively and initiating investigations prior to medical assessment, providing postoperative care and contraceptive advice at clinics
Minor surgery	Performing pre- and postoperative assessment of patients, accepting direct referrals and performing minor surgery under local anaesthetic

Numerous articles, newspaper reports and documents from various national associations have discussed the need to ensure that post holders are appropriately trained, that clinical duties should only be delegated if they are within the scope of the post holder's skills, that patients must be aware that non-medical staff are involved in their care and that supervision is provided.

The Royal College of Surgeons and the Royal College of Nursing have undertaken an investigation of the unstructured developments which have taken place so far and identified a way forward. This work was published as a discussion document in September 1999 and is entitled *Assistants in surgical practice*. The NATN document *Developing new roles for non-medical staff within perioperative care. Guidelines for organisations and employers* (NATN 1997) provides excellent guidance for those intending to set up new roles.

Specific guidelines for heads of department where cardiac surgeons' assistants are being appointed were produced in 1994 by the Royal College of Surgeons and the Society of Cardiothoracic Surgeons. These were designed to set standards for education and parameters of responsibility and to ensure a satisfactory service for patients, allowing for flexibility and local initiatives. Currently, the training for cardiac surgeon's assistant is 2 years although students are eligible to take the RCS final assessment at 1 year if they are recommended by the consultant surgeon supervising their training. However, trainees will not receive the RCS certificate until they have completed 2 full years of practice as a cardiac surgeon's assistant.

In Manchester, a module of the BSc(Hons) Nursing/Midwifery Practice entitled *The nurse practitioner in perioperative care* (ENB D10) has been approved to further develop nurses who have completed the N77. In other centres, NVQ competencies for surgical assistants have been used to underpin the training programme. The fact that training is provided at local level has resulted in a lack of transferability. A national training programme with core elements for all surgical assistants is preferable.

One of the key issues when developing a new role, especially that of surgeon's assistant where invasive procedures may be undertaken, is for doctors, non-medical personnel and managers to work closely together to plan the development in a structured manner and to take note of the impact such a development may have. Seeking advice from the regulatory bodies or professional associations may be appropriate and visiting centres which have already established a post is most worthwhile.

The anaesthetist's assistant/nurse anaesthetist

The need for anaesthetic assistants or nurse anaesthetists has been under debate and the parameters for any such role have not been defined. The degrees of independence afforded to such a practitioner, the levels of supervision and lines of command will need to be defined if these posts should ever develop.

The Royal College of Anaesthetists recommend that personnel assisting the anaesthetist must undergo a minimum of 6 months supernumerary training. The Association of Anaesthetists of Great Britain and Ireland (AAGBI) and the Royal College of Anaesthetists (RCA) have both indicated their strong support for creating a body of trained assistants for anaesthetists. These two bodies produced *Anaesthesia in Great Britain and Ireland. A physician only service* (1996) which stressed the need for skilled assistants. If appropriate levels of assistance for anaesthetists are not provided, the Royal College of Anaesthetists can remove training accreditation from hospitals.

The role of the nurse or ODP during anaesthesia is to assist in the preparation, maintenance and monitoring of anaesthesia and the care of the anaesthetised patient. The assistants do not administer general anaesthesia. This differs from the role of the nurse anaesthetist which has emerged in the USA and some European countries. Nurse anaesthetists undergo additional training which allows them to induce, maintain and reverse general anaesthesia. In the USA, the certificated registered nurse anaesthetist (CRNA) is a recognised advanced practice role and there is strong impetus for the minimum preparation for advanced practice roles to be a Master's degree (Hodson 1998). The CRNA role also includes preoperative assessment and following through postoperative instructions. The CRNA can practise independently but this varies between centres depending on the physician anaesthetist support available. The RCA and AAGBI do not support the development of such a role; anaesthesia in Great Britain and Ireland is exclusively a medical speciality.

In the UK training to assist the anaesthetist is part of the basic ODP programme. Nurses have to access either the ODP anaesthetic competencies or a National Board approved anaesthetic course after their basic training and after a period of employment in the operating department. It is therefore more common to see ODPs assisting the anaesthetist but with the short supply of theatre staff and the need for flexible staffing and multiskilling, support for anaesthetists can be of a variable standard. To this end, *Professional roles in anaesthetics: a scoping study* (Reilly et al 1996) was published by the NHS Executive to establish the best way of supporting anaesthetists. The issue of nurse anaesthetists was debated within the remit of the study. Some of the recommendations from the study were as follows.

• Trusts should be encouraged to avoid ad hoc developments which involve a significant adjustment of professional roles in the anaesthetic service in order to cope with the current workforce shortage.

• There is obvious scope for the adjustment of professional roles within the anaesthetic service as demonstrated by the considerable variation in professional roles identified in the study. Trusts which have successfully adjusted roles and evaluated them to the benefit of patient care and professional developments in existing service areas should be identified and used as models of good practice.

• The concept of the anaesthetic team should be further explored and developed.

• A unified grade of operating department support staff providing anaesthetic assistance in the operating theatre should be reconsidered. The role and career structure of such a grade should be clarified and formalised within clearly defined parameters. Entry to such a grade should be open to nurses and ODPs. There is a need for a coherent and unified educational strategy for theatre staff and future courses should capitalise on the strength of existing courses. Qualifications should be accredited. The national Nursing Education Board should seek to ensure nursing qualifications receive UK-wide recognition.

• Workforce planning for the anaesthetic team, including operating department and ITU medical and non-medical staff, should be explored and relate closely to business plans and purchaser intentions.

Pilot sites were set up, closely monitored by the Department of Health, RCA and AAGBI, to take forward initiatives which may adjust professional roles within the anaesthetic service. This study has been completed and the report is in preparation. The AAGBI jointly with the RCA is also considering how best involvement of non-medical personnel in the operating department can be progressed and have published a document entitled *The anaesthetic team* (1998).

Other roles associated with perioperative practice

The numerous new roles emerging in the health service have many titles. Non-medical personnel have taken on activities previously carried out by medical staff, as described above, and it is quite possible that their roles do not fit into the definitions of first or surgical assistant but that they do contribute to perioperative care. Titles which have been assumed to describe the developing roles of nurses include clinical nurse specialist, nurse practitioner, specialist practitioner and advanced practitioner. Concern is frequently expressed in the literature about what these titles mean.

The UKCC (1994) definitions of specialist and advanced practitioner, as specified in its document on education and practice following registration, were clear and were associated with study at graduate and Master's level as well as enhanced practice. However, these titles are being used in ways which do not relate to the UKCC definitions. In an effort to clarify the situation and set standards within the postregistration regulatory framework, the UKCC agreed not to set standards for advanced practice but to support the notion of advancing practice (UKCC 1997). A framework which would embrace existing nurse specialists/practitioners would be explored and consultation work was commenced (UKCC 1998). In the meantime, new roles with unclear titles remain and only discussion with the post holder and examination of the job description will illustrate the parameters of such roles. New standards for the UKCC Higher Level Practice Registration will be piloted during 1999 and 2000.

There is, therefore, no way to clarify how such post holders may contribute to perioperative care but Box 9.3 gives a few examples.

Box 9.3 Possible contributions to perioperative care	
Preadmission clinics	Preparing patients for surgical admission
Nurse-led day surgery units	Assessing patients for surgery, assisting in the operating theatre and providing postoperative care and advice
Critical care practitioners	Providing postoperative care after surgery in the recovery/critical care environment. This may include prescribing treatment within protocols
Clinician's assistants	Assessing and preparing patients for transplant surgery, coordination of the recipient operation and postoperative care and counselling

Many specialities may also have nurses who undertake pre- and postoperative assessment of patients, order investigations and act as a first assistant in theatre if required. Others may be appointed to provide a specific aspect of patient care such as stoma care or pain management.

Principles to consider when developing roles for non-medical personnel in perioperative practice

The principles which should be considered when developing the roles of non-medical staff within perioperative care are:

- parameters of new roles;
- education and training;
- professional implications;
- managerial and personnel issues;
- legal and ethical issues.

These principles have already been discussed in great detail elsewhere (NATN 1993, 1994, 1997) and are not covered further in this chapter.

The haphazard way in which new roles have developed and the fact that the parameters of roles are set at a local level make explicit job profiles essential. These should be reviewed on a regular basis. If additional practice is added to an existing post this should also be expressed within the job profile.

For the purpose of clinical risk management all disciplines should consider the potential impact of non-medical staff taking on activities which were previously carried out by medical staff. Patient safety is of paramount importance and the essential elements of training and assessment must be addressed.

Dowling et al (1996) identified considerable confusion regarding accountability within new role development. Post holders have to work across three areas of regulation: the professional regulations of the UKCC and the General Medical Council (GMC); civil law; and employment law. Post holders and employers must be fully versed in the potential professional and legal implications of any developments they introduce.

Personnel and managerial implications have to be explored. Salary grading has to be considered and developing a new role may not be the most cost-effective option. The future career pathway for post holders should also be considered before appointments are made.

CONCERNS ABOUT THE DEVELOPMENT OF NEW ROLES

The ad hoc way in which new roles have developed in various specialities means that there is no national register recording such developments. There are no national standards for training staff to undertake new activities and there is no central monitoring process. Throughout the UK, regional task forces for junior doctors' hours have pump-primed new posts which were created specifically to reduce the hours of junior doctors. Apart from a few centres, it appears that the introduction of these posts and the use of vast amounts of NHS money have not been monitored. It would be interesting to explore how many such posts still exist to evaluate why some posts succeeded and others did not. In light of the new health service agenda of clinical effectiveness, more time should perhaps be spent measuring the outcomes of these new roles.

It is essential throughout the process of promoting team work and developing new roles that junior doctors' training is not compromised. The service commitment of training grades has been reduced since the Calman Report (1993) and it is therefore important to ensure that the opportunities they have for learning in the clinical areas are maximised.

The emergence of a new 'elitist', higher tier of non-medical staff has produced disparities in monetary rewards, titles, training, registration and career pathways. The opportunity to undertake new roles and duties may not be available to all non-medical staff or desired by all. Whilst some may consider that new role development assists with recruitment and retention by allowing staff to develop, the opposite effect could be true. As the 'elitist' tier of staff taking on new duties get paid more or are seen to be 'special', the foundation core of non-medical staff must also be rewarded in some way otherwise there is a danger that they will become disenchanted and look elsewhere for employment.

Time also has to be spent considering the overall staffing picture. As health-care professionals move into new roles, who does the job that they used to do? Nationally there is a major shortage of health-care professionals, especially in the operating department. Whilst the short-term answer may be to train unqualified staff to do more, the long-term solution is still unclear.

Many of the key principles discussed in this chapter are not being considered before new posts are created. In particular, time should be spent ensuring that parameters of roles are clear and documented within the job profile, that education and training are provided and, where possible, this training is nationally transferable. An assessment process for post holders should be provided and this should include what happens if an employee fails an assessment. Employers and employees need to consider the relevant legal, ethical and professional issues. Personnel officers and managers have to discuss terms and conditions of employment, grading and career progression.

For many years there has been debate on whether qualified nurses are required in the operating room. If perioperative nurses move away from their traditional roles to undertake tasks previously done by junior doctors, they may be accused of writing their own obituary in the operating room.

CONCLUSION

It is apparent that the UKCC's *Scope of professional practice* (1992) and the need to reduce junior doctors' hours have been major catalysts in the development of team working and new roles.

Many papers illustrate the background to these developments and some studies have explored the merits or otherwise of non-medical staff undertaking tasks which were previously the preserve of doctors. However, the ad hoc manner in which new roles have developed and the lack of any national register or training standard continue to cause concern. Further work exploring the outcomes of new role development is essential.

There is increasing pressure within the health service to evaluate developments and provide evidence of effectiveness. However, there is little academic work specifically evaluating the role of the surgical assistant. National studies have been commissioned to explore the merits of new roles in general, but none focuses solely on roles which have developed for non-medical staff within perioperative care.

The introduction of clinical governance will put a great deal of emphasis on continuing professional development and on evidence of competence. Non-medical staff who have taken on new activities must be seen to maintain their competence. As skills are cascaded throughout a professional group, non-medical staff must ensure that they practise frequently enough to maintain their skills and delegating medical staff should periodically verify competence.

The reduction in the amount of service time provided by doctors in training continues to be high on the health service agenda. This means that many of the activities which are currently new to non-medical personnel will in time become the norm and training for such activities should be included in preregistration programmes. However, if new areas of training are added to the basic nurse training curriculum, what, if anything, can be removed from the traditional syllabus? Many nurse tutors would argue that the syllabus is already too full without adding more competencies.

Finally, the shortage of perioperative staff is a national problem. The number of nurses and practitioners entering the profession is declining and whilst enhancing practice may in the short term aid recruitment and retention, there are no long-term solutions. In the future, questions have to be asked about who will staff operating departments. From which backgrounds will these staff come? What qualifications will they need? What are the essential skills that they will need? How will their activities be monitored and regulated? Whatever the answers, operating department staff will need to work flexibly as a team to provide the best possible care for the patient.

REFERENCES

AAGBI, RCA 1996 Anaesthesia in Great Britain and Ireland. A physician only service. AAGBI and RCA, London
AAGBI, RCA 1998 The anaesthetic team. AAGBI and RCA, London
Association of Operating Room Nurses 1984 AORN official statement on RN first assistants. AORN Journal 40: 3
Audit Commission 1995 The doctors' tale. The work of hospital doctors in England and Wales. HMSO, London

Bevan P G 1989 The management and utilisation of operating departments. NHSME, London

Calman K 1993 Hospital doctors: training for the future. The report of the working group on specialist medical training. Department of Health, London

Dowling S, Martin R, Skidmore P, Doyal L, Cameron A, Lloyd S 1996 Nurses taking on junior doctors' work. A confusion of accountability. British Medical Journal 312: 1211–1214

Greenhalgh & Co 1994 The interface between junior doctors and nurses – research study for the Department of Health. Greenhalgh & Co, Macclesfield

Hodson D 1998 The evolving role of advanced nurses in surgery. AORN Journal 67: 5

King's Fund 1997 Exploring new roles in practice (ENRiP) database. King's Fund, London

Levenson R, Vaughan B 1999 Developing new roles in practice: an evidence-based guide. SCHARR, University of Sheffield

NATN 1993 The role of the nurse as first assistant in the operating department. National Association of Theatre Nurses, Harrogate

NATN 1994 The nurse as surgeon's assistant. National Association of Theatre Nurses, Harrogate

NATN 1996 The role of the support worker. National Association of Theatre Nurses, Harrogate

NATN 1997 Developing new roles for non medical staff within perioperative care. Guidelines for organisations and employers. National Association of Theatre Nurses, Harrogate

NHS Centre for Reviews and Dissemination 1997 Practice and service development. Anglia and Oxford Database of Practice and Service Developments, York

NHS Management Executive 1991 Junior doctors: the new deal. NHSME, London

Read S 1995 Catching the tide: new voyages in nursing? SCHARR occasional paper no. 1. SCHARR, Sheffield

Read S, Graves K 1994 Reduction of junior doctors' hours in Trent Region: the nursing contribution. NHS Executive, Sheffield

Reilly C, Challands A, Barrett A, Read S 1996 Professional roles in anaesthetics: a scoping study. NHS Executive, Leeds

Rothrock J 1987 A college without walls. Learning first assistant skills. AORN Journal 45: 5

Royal College of Surgeons of England 1991 Assistants in surgical practice. RCS, London

Royal College of Surgeons and Society of Cardiothoracic Surgeons 1994 Cardiac surgeon's assistants. Guidelines for heads of department. RCS and SCS, London

Scottish Office Department of Health, National Nursing, Midwifery and Health Visiting Advisory Committee 1995a Health service developments and the scope of professional nursing practice. A survey of pertinent literature. Scottish Office, Edinburgh

Scottish Office Department of Health, National Nursing, Midwifery and Health Visiting Advisory Committee 1995b Health service developments and the scope of professional nursing practice. A survey of developing clinical roles within NHS trusts in Scotland. Scottish Office, Edinburgh

Touche Ross & Co 1994 Evaluation of nurse practitioner pilot projects. South Thames RHA/NHS Executive, London

UKCC 1992 The scope of professional practice. United Kingdom Central Council, London

UKCC 1994 The council's standards for education and practice following registration. United Kingdom Central Council, London

UKCC 1997 Press statement (8/97). United Kingdom Central Council, London

UKCC 1998 A higher level of practice. Consultation document. United Kingdom Central Council, London

United Kingdom Health Departments, Joint Consultants Committee and Chairmen of Regional Health Authorities 1987 Hospital medical staffing: achieving a balance. HMSO, London

FURTHER READING

Coopers & Lybrand 1996 Nurse practitioner evaluation project. Final report. NHS Management Executive, Leeds

Dimond B 1994 Legal aspects of role expansion. In: Hunt G, Wainwright P (eds) Expanding the role of the nurse – the scope of professional practice. Blackwell, Oxford

Dowling S, Barrett S, West R 1995 With nurse practitioners, who needs house officers? British Medical Journal 311: 309–313

Hunt G, Wainwright P (eds) 1994 Expanding the role of the nurse – the scope of professional practice. Blackwell, Oxford

Evidence-based practice in the perioperative environment

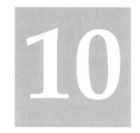

Marion Taylor

'Evidence-based practice' – is this just the latest fad in the NHS, nothing but the latest phase in health-care provision, current management buzz-words which are irrelevant to clinical practice? Or is it something that really matters? Something that all perioperative staff need to be aware of and involved in? The answer is, of course, the latter.

Staff working in the perioperative environment need to consider, understand and make moves towards evidence-based practice. It is not an easy concept, it is not easy to do in the real-life, busy world of operating departments and it cannot be implemented overnight. It is much easier to carry on doing things 'the way we've always done them'. Evidence-based practice takes more effort, commitment and understanding but it needs to be addressed in every operating department in the country. This chapter aims to assist the perioperative practitioner with both the concept and the practicality of evidence-based practice.

UNDERSTANDING EVIDENCE-BASED PRACTICE

Nurses working in the perioperative environment are required to keep up to date in their professional practice for many reasons. These include the *Code of professional conduct, Guidelines for professional practice* and PREP requirements for registration. There is also the increased expectation for nurses to develop research-based care and to keep abreast of all important research findings.

There have been wide-ranging developments in many areas in the perioperative environment, including, for example, the amount and complexity of technology being used, rapid anaesthetic and surgical developments, expanding and changing roles, nurses taking on aspects of care previously identified as 'doctors' work' and the development of increasingly narrow surgical specialisms. Also, all staff involved in health-care provision now encounter a general public with high expectations of their health-care system. This is influenced by an increase in the public's awareness, interest and knowledge of health-related issues, an increased awareness of their rights and treatments and an increase in liability claims and legal actions for medical negligence, as discussed in Chapter 7. Nurses therefore have a responsibility to ensure that they give clinically effective care, based on the best possible evidence.

These contributing factors and many other changes within the health services have influenced the development of evidence-based practice within medicine and, more recently, nursing. The term 'evidence-based practice' (EBP) has been used since about 1995 and now has a range of literature and journals to support it. However, a clear explanation of what the term means has not always been provided. It may therefore have been perceived as being the same as conducting/implementing research, something that is only relevant for medical staff or those working in academia or clinical research.

While EBP is linked to all these aspects, they do not tell the whole story; thus a definition is useful. Evidence-based practice can be defined as 'an approach to decision making in which the clinician uses the best evidence available' (Gray 1997). There are many such definitions in the literature, each of which highlights another facet of EBP, and as this movement began in medicine, a definition from there is useful to understand the origins of the terminology. Sackett et al (1996) define EBP as the 'conscientious, explicit and judicious use of current best evidence about the care of an individual patient'. EBP has emerged from this and incorporates all aspects of health-care provision, of which nursing is an essential part.

A final thought on definitions comes from Thompson (1998), who suggests that 'Evidence-based health care, including nursing, is about incorporating research evidence with clinical expertise, the resources available and the views of the patients'. This is both helpful and practical and highlights how EBP involves much more than research: the views of both clinicians and patients are also relevant and the necessary implications of resources are also recognised. This is supported by Walsh (1998), who also identifies the difficulties inherent in using patient satisfaction evidence.

Perioperative EBP therefore involves nurses:

- adopting an approach to perioperative care in which individuals are aware of their actions;
- questioning day-to-day practices;
- being open and receptive to changes in practice;
- being aware of the importance of research;
- being able to critically appraise and incorporate evidence into their practice when appropriate.

It does not mean that all practitioners should be doing research, producing evidence, writing and publishing but that they should use evidence to assist them to identify best practices for patient care. Managers therefore need to ensure that the working environment is conducive to this and that systems are in place to incorporate evidence into everyday practice.

EBP therefore represents a broader way of looking at practice than the carrying out or the utilisation of research and incorporates the concept of clinical effectiveness as outlined in Chapters 5 and 6. The terms associated with EBP are defined in Box 10.1.

Box 10.1   Useful terms

1. **Evidence-based medicine** – the conscientious, explicit and judicious use of current best evidence about the care of an individual patient (Sackett et al 1996)
2. **Evidence-based nursing** – is about incorporating research evidence with clinical expertise, the resources available and the views of the patients (Thompson 1998)
3. **Evidence-based practice** – an approach to decision making in which the clinician uses the best evidence available (Gray 1997)
4. **Clinical effectiveness** – the extent to which specific clinical interventions, when deployed in the field for a particular patient or population, do what they are intended to do, i.e. maintain and improve health and secure the greatest possible health gain from the available resources (NHSE 1996a)
5. **Clinical governance** – a mechanism by which trust boards and chief executives are ultimately responsible for the effectiveness and clinical quality of work carried out within the trust (Fennessey 1998)
6. **Clinical audit** – a process whereby clinicians examine their practices and results against agreed standards and modify their practice where indicated (NHSE 1996c)
7. **Clinical guidelines** – systematically developed statements designed to assist clinicians and patients make decisions about appropriate treatment for specific conditions. They are published and maintained by professional bodies, e.g. the investigation and treatment of stable angina, the management of acute low back pain (NHSE 1996b)
8. **Systematic review** – in this process all the research on a clinical intervention is systematically sought, appraised and assessed for rigour, reliability and validity and an overview of the collated findings is made (Nursing and Midwifery Audit Service 1998)
9. **Meta-analysis** – this comprehensively identifies all the literature on a topic and also incorporates a specific statistical strategy for accumulating the results of several studies into a single estimate (Sackett et al 1991)
10. **Quality assurance** – taking positive action to assess and evaluate performance against agreed defined standards in order to create and manage a service which regularly achieves desired levels of care or service (Ball 1989)
11. **Standard** – a statement which outlines an objective with guidance for its achievement given in the form of required resources, activities and predicted outcomes (RCN 1990)

The impetus for EBP came in the mid 1990s when the Department of Health set up a task force, headed by Sir Anthony Culyer, to discover how the research it commissioned was being implemented and disseminated. One finding of this report was that clinical decision making is rarely based on any evidence but more often on the practitioner's personal judgement (Culyer 1995). In order to address this, systematic reviews of research were advocated; these are defined in Box 10.1.

Research evidence can be found in different publications, requiring a literature search before reviewing and appraising the evidence. A systematic review allows practitioners to short cut this step. Within the UK the NHS Research and Development Directorate has identified two centres of excellence that conduct systematic reviews:

- NHS Centre for Reviews and Dissemination at the University of York;
- UK Cochrane Centre, Oxford.

Abstracts of these centres' work are available on CD-ROM:

- Database of Abstracts of Reviews and Effectiveness – DARE;
- Cochrane Library.

They are also available as the publications *Effectiveness matters* and *Effective health care bulletins*. Other sources of systematic reviews are:

- the King's Fund Developments Programme;
- RCN Institute Dynamic Quality Improvement Programme;
- RCN Nursing and Midwifery Audit Information Service;
- St George's Hospital, London;
- Scottish Intercollegiate Network (SIGN).

Details on these are given at the end of the chapter.

The major developments in EBP are shown in Box 10.2. This is useful to highlight how recently the EBP movement began but also how rapidly it is progressing.

The centres in York and Oxford therefore offer easy access to EBP; all the research has been appraised and recommendations made for practice. Evidence-based nursing, as we shall see, is more difficult. Most of the reviews performed so far have been on scientific experimental studies, not the messy real-life stuff of nursing and perioperative practice. Most

---

Box 10.2   Development of evidence-based practice

1991   Department of Health strategy launched – *Research for health*. This aimed to create a knowledge-based health service in which clinical, managerial and policy decisions are based on sound information about research findings and scientific development (DoH 1991).

1992   Task force set up, headed by Sir Anthony Culyer, to discover how research was being commissioned, implemented and disseminated.

1995   The task force reported – the Culyer Report (1995).

1996   *Promoting clinical effectiveness – a framework for action in and through the NHS* published by the NHSE.

1997   Research and development *towards an evidence-based health service* (DoH 1997).

1997   Implementation of *Clinical effectiveness* initiatives by the NHSE.

1998   Implementation of RCN's *Clinical effectiveness initiatives*.

1998   *Evidence-Based Nursing* journal published.

nursing research is qualitative and involves relatively small unicentre samples, in contrast with the multicentre randomised controlled trials (RCTs) of medicine.

Moreover, perioperative practice is further complicated by the multiprofessional teamwork involved in anaesthetic and surgical practice. While this teamwork provides an excellent environment for staff to work in and an appropriate mix of skills to care for the patient, it makes for a difficult area for research. The complexities of surgical practice are also influenced by others caring for the surgical patient in the extended team – including ward staff and through infection control practices, for example.

Why should evidence-based care be practised?

Most importantly, this approach to everyday practice should be used to benefit the patients. Heater et al (1988) report that patients who receive research-based nursing care make a sizeable gain in behavioural knowledge, physiological and psychological outcomes, compared to those receiving routine nursing care. Smith (1997) also relates the need for evidence-based care to the *Code of professional conduct* and *Guidelines for professional practice* and identifies that nurses have a responsibility to ensure that the care they give patients is based on the best possible evidence.

In order to identify why evidence-based care should be practised in the perioperative environment, it is helpful to consider the alternatives. Examples of care that are not based on evidence come from both medicine and nursing. Lewis (1993) identifies that in England about 49 000 women under 40 years of age have a dilation and curettage operation, despite this procedure being of little therapeutic value – it simply does not achieve its aims. Walsh & Ford (1989) provide many examples of nursing rituals of no clinical use and that sometimes even harm and Wicker (1997) provides examples of other rituals or 'sacred cows' in the perioperative environment. Practices not based on evidence must therefore be based on something else.

- Personal choice and preference of the individual care givers (these may vary greatly): for example, masks being worn for some surgeons' lists but not for others'.
- The practice of another person – a role model. Again, this can vary greatly and may often be poor practice; for example, some theatre staff scrubbing for 3 minutes, some for 5 minutes.
- Ritual, 'it's always been done that way', custom and practice: for example, nil by mouth times.
- Financial considerations: for example, some patients receiving a preoperative visit from theatre staff and others not, when it is too busy.
- Out-of-date or inadequate research findings.
- Policies or procedure documents that are out of date or inconsistent.

- Recommendations by someone with a vested interest, such as an individual who has researched the topic personally or a commercial company, for example.

Perioperative care that is not evidence based will therefore be inconsistent, vary according to who is on duty, be difficult to explain to others as there is no knowledge base, may be done because it is the cheapest option and is unlikely to provide the patient with the best possible care. In contrast, perioperative care that is based on evidence should:

- be of the same standard all the time, regardless of who provides the care;
- be able to be explained by knowledge, research and experience;
- be up to date;
- be based on quality of care as well as financial considerations;
- form the basis of any policies, procedures, clinical practice guidelines, standard setting and audit tools used.

Students, juniors and staff new to the operating department often trigger the consideration of practice by more senior staff by asking 'Why is that done that way?' and asking for further information on something, thus identifying EBP, or the lack of it, as the following two extracts from newly qualified staff nurses' reflective journals show.

Case study 10.1   Evidence-based practice?

We spent so much time doing these reflective journals as students I don't seem to be able to stop now I'm qualified! Mind you, I feel like a student, being a new staff nurse in the operating department certainly makes me aware of just how junior I am, and how much I've got to learn.

Today was good, I'm still asking loads of questions – another flash-back to being a student, but the staff don't seem to mind so long as I pick the right moment.

The sister I'm working with is interested in my questions at the moment, as she's one of the group updating the policy book for the department – a really big project, and she says my questions serve as a prompt for her to find some 'evidence'.

I asked her to explain. Evidence she says is some information that is so strong and so good that it affects the way you care for the patients, and the written policies that explain this to all the staff.

There are some good pieces of evidence to use in operating departments, *Safeguards for invasive procedures: the management of risks* (NATN et al 1998) for example, which states how to check patients into the operating department and how to do swab counts. I was initially a bit confused: 'But it's not research, is it?' I asked. Sister explained, no, but it was a set of national guidelines, written by a group of national experts, who have agreed on these guidelines. She explained that 'evidence' can come in many forms, of which research was only one. We discussed other national guidelines that influence our practice, but are

Case study 10.1 cont.

not research – the *Code of conduct*, health and safety law, EC directives, UKCC documents, for example.

'What about proper research, we are using it, aren't we?' I asked, having spent 3 years writing academic essays about the importance of it. She explained that, yes, we do use it when we can, when it exists, is available and is of good quality, but that using it is not always easy. 'I thought you just found a good paper, read it, and implemented the changes.' Sister looked shocked, 'No, no, no and no!'; as she told me more, I began to understand that the research has to be critically evaluated and, if it is appropriate, then the long haul of implementing the change begins, so that all staff do the same – not as easy as I thought!

Furthermore, there are some bits of evidence that are very difficult to find – one of my questions that prompted her was 'Why does everyone scrub up differently, for different lengths of time, using different techniques?'. I had tried asking a few people this and was met with the 'I've always done it this way' type of answer. Sister said it is a difficult one and one which we will tackle together – we're going to the library tomorrow to start our literature search – as I've asked the question I have to help! Maybe now I can see the attraction of 'always doing it this way!' Still, I really feel like I'm learning, I'm grasping this evidence-based practice I think, and think I'm helping as well.

Case study 10.2   Or not?

I know I don't have to continue with this journal now I'm qualified, but I thought I'd keep it up as things are so difficult at the moment. I seem to be doing everything wrong, writing it down might make things a bit clearer. Today was difficult, although a typical day since I began in theatres 2 weeks ago. I know I'm new and probably stupid and I've got so much to learn, I just wish someone would help me.

I've tried to ask my questions at the right times, when it's quiet or we're just waiting around. It's just so difficult to get any answers, I've tried my mentor, the sister in the theatre, even a doctor, but I'm not getting any answers, so it's really difficult to learn. Whatever I've asked the answers are a variation on a theme.

'We've always done it this way.'

'It's the policy.'

'Sister says to do it this way.'

'Mr Adams likes it this way', etc., etc.

Such similar answers to such a variety of questions.

'Why does everyone scrub differently? Should I scrub my hands with the brush or just my nails?'

'Why do they use different drapes in orthopaedics?'

'Why do we wear masks for some things and not others?'

They all refer to 'the policies' quite a lot but I can't find them. Apparently they are locked in the office to stop them getting lost – no wonder we can't use them.

Anyway, I think I'll stop asking questions now, I seem to be getting on everyone's nerves. It's just that as students we were taught and expected to

Case study 10.2 cont.
ask questions and find out information for ourselves. My friend say that on
her ward they're starting to implement something called 'evidence-based
practice'. I wonder what that is.

Reviewing your practice and identifying problems in practice

The impetus for changing practice should have its origins in the wish to
address a problem and improve practice, rather than merely for the sake
of change. Such problems may be apparent and obvious to you.

- The department policy for MRSA patients is not practical and thus not
  followed.
- Staff in your department feel it is acceptable to wear jewellery in theatre.
- Patients' dignity and privacy within a large recovery room are
  sometimes compromised.

Real-life problems such as these within your department should provide
priorities for you to address. If you are not aware of such practice-based
problems you either work in a perfect department or you need to review
your practice further. This can be achieved by considering the effects of
your perioperative practice on others – namely your patients. For this,
many problem indicators can be used.

- Infection rates within surgical specialities.
- Incidence of pressure sore development in surgical patients.
- Cancellation rates.
- Incidence of errors in surgical practice.
- Incidence of recovery room closing.

Trusts will each have a variety of means for capturing such data – quality
assurance, standards, audits, etc. – and these can provide a useful source of
information about areas of perioperative practice that can be improved. Also
consider ideas from other staff: for example, the manager, at staff meetings,
students who have placements within the department, medical staff, infection
control group or the tissue viability/wound management group.

Reviewing your practice therefore means considering your daily work
and then identifying a topic for tackling on the basis of EBP. What is
good? What is not good? What could be improved? Tackling any change
in practice is not something that can usually be done alone, so enlist some
help and the support (in principle at least) of your manager.

Finding the evidence – search tools

Once a particular problem/area of practice has been identified, the next
step is to find the best evidence available. One difficult practical (and
possibly ethical) problem with implementing EBP is that an individual's
access to the evidence will vary according to:

- place of work (e.g. district general hospital, teaching hospital, private sector, etc.);
- infrastructure of the institution (research activity, practice development strategies, etc.);
- access to library facilities;
- extent of the library facilities, search tools available, journals held, etc.

The aim of EBP is to implement the best evidence available to you and traditionally this would have involved undertaking a literature search. Recently, however, this has become a more difficult task, with the huge increase in both published research and the number of journals. Most nursing/medical libraries now offer a system of literature searching using CD-ROM databases. These are computer indexes such as CINAHL (Cumulative Index to Nursing and Allied Health Literature) and Medline. Librarians will be able to assist those new to this type of literature searching and further information is given on this at the end of this section.

The second part of literature searching is critically reviewing the journal articles obtained. This involves considering the recommendations made in a piece of research and deciding whether they should be implemented within your department or not. There are many books and journal articles that can help the reader with this process and examples are included in the Further reading section.

A review of research findings is therefore helpful for clinical staff who not have the time, facilities or skills to undertake such an activity. A systematic review is defined as 'the process of systematically locating, appraising and synthesising evidence from scientific studies in order to obtain a reliable overview' (NHS Centre for Reviews and Dissemination 1996). This then is a useful tool, as clinical staff can be assured that all the relevant research has been obtained and that it has been rigorously appraised.

A further process involved in the review of evidence is a 'meta-analysis'. This activity considers data from a range of studies incorporating RCTs and applies a range of statistical techniques (McMahon 1997), in order to make recommendations for practice. Access to these systematic reviews is by CD-ROM in a nursing or medical library. Steps have also been made to increase dissemination of this evidence in the journal *Evidence-Based Nursing*, which provides systematic reviews and recommendations on a variety of nursing topics. The *Nursing Standard* (1997) has also published a compilation of reviews relevant to nursing.

- Non-pharmacological interventions for acute pain.
- Use of compression stockings.
- The prevention and treatment of pressure sores.
- Preventing falls and further injury in older people.
- Preoperative patient instruction: is it effective?
- Use of nasogastric tubes for effective laparotomy.
- Managing primary breast cancer: a review of care.
- Psychoeducational care for adults with cancer.
- Psychosocial interventions for coronary artery disease.

These provide a definitive overview of research to date on each topic but for the majority of nursing topics, including most aspects of perioperative practice, there is no systematic review of evidence available at present, although this is a rapidly evolving area.

Where, then, does this leave perioperative staff who wish to develop EBP? They may have access to influence and support from other members of the team, but a lack of systematic reviews on relevant areas of practice. Evidence can still be used but it will be evidence of a different type.

Quality of evidence/grading scales/rating the evidence

Morgan & Fennessey (1996) have developed the concept of 'levels of evidence', which identifies the wide variety of evidence that can be used. Perioperative staff must therefore be aware of what evidence they are basing their practice on. This is useful at different stages: first, when considering present policies – what are they based on? Second, when implementing new evidence to improve practice – what type of evidence is it? Figure 10.1 shows the Morgan & Fennessey (1996) levels of evidence, and Figure 10.2 shows a simplified form of this by Thompson & Cullum (1999).

Within the perioperative environment there are a great deal of primary research studies – the effects of mask wearing, the effects of preoperative visiting, for example – but there are few instances of research that has been collated, reviewed and disseminated as guidelines for practice.

There are also many areas of practice that are based on expert opinion or accepted practice and this is likely to be the case for some time, until a 'higher' level of evidence, such as a systematic review, is available. Lack of a systematic review therefore does not mean that the care being practised is of poor quality or is not based on any evidence but that the evidence may be of a lower level and theatre practitioners should be aware of this.

It is possible to raise awareness of the type of evidence in use by considering areas of practice and identifying what they are based on. An aspect of perioperative practice based on guidelines from a recognised nursing body may not have included a systematic review of the evidence but is based on a wide view of expert opinion. Documents such as the *Principles of safe practice in the perioperative environment* (NATN 1998) fall into this category of evidence. Perioperative staff should therefore use the best evidence available to them but with insight and understanding of the type of evidence it is. They should also be aware of the development of higher level evidence and understand the significance of systematic reviews/meta-analyses when they become available.

Reading the evidence – critical evaluation

Once a literature search has obtained evidence relevant to the area of practice you wish to change, it is necessry to review, read and critically evaluate it. The first part of this is the consideration of the type of evidence and this is followed by a 'critique' or 'critical evaluation' of the

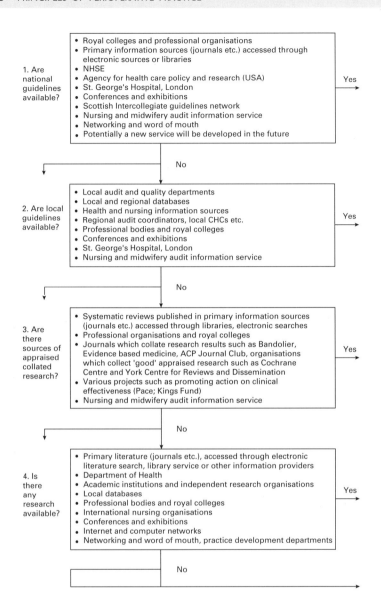

Figure 10.1 Levels of evidence (Morgan & Fennessey 1996).

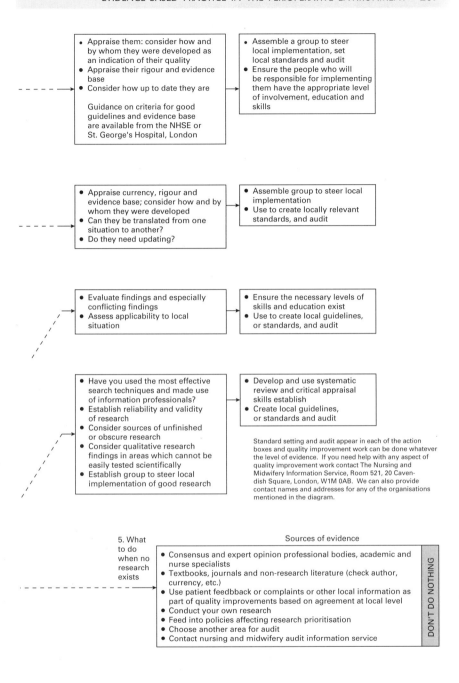

- Appraise them: consider how and by whom they were developed as an indication of their quality
- Appraise their rigour and evidence base
- Consider how up to date they are

  Guidance on criteria for good guidelines and evidence base are available from the NHSE or St. George's Hospital, London

- Assemble a group to steer local implementation, set local standards and audit
- Ensure the people who will be responsible for implementing them have the appropriate level of involvement, education and skills

- Appraise currency, rigour and evidence base; consider how and by whom they were developed
- Can they be translated from one situation to another?
- Do they need updating?

- Assemble group to steer local implementation
- Use to create locally relevant standards, and audit

- Evaluate findings and especially conflicting findings
- Assess applicability to local situation

- Ensure the necessary levels of skills and education exist
- Use to create local guidelines, or standards, and audit

- Have you used the most effective search techniques and made use of information professionals?
- Establish reliability and validity of research
- Consider sources of unfinished or obscure research
- Consider qualitative research findings in areas which cannot be easily tested scientifically
- Establish group to steer local implementation of good research

- Develop and use systematic review and critical appraisal skills establish
- Create local guidelines, or standards and audit

Standard setting and audit appear in each of the action boxes and quality improvement work can be done whatever the level of evidence. If you need help with any aspect of quality improvement work contact The Nursing and Midwifery Information Service, Room 521, 20 Cavendish Square, London, W1M 0AB. We can also provide contact names and addresses for any of the organisations mentioned in the diagram.

5. What to do when no research exists

Sources of evidence

- Consensus and expert opinion professional bodies, academic and nurse specialists
- Textbooks, journals and non-research literature (check author, currency, etc.)
- Use patient feedbback or complaints or other local information as part of quality improvements based on agreement at local level
- Conduct your own research
- Feed into policies affecting research prioritisation
- Choose another area for audit
- Contact nursing and midwifery audit information service

DON'T DO NOTHING

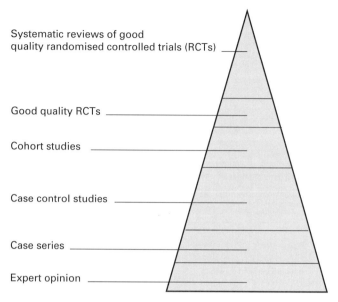

Figure 10.2   Simplified levels of evidence (Thompson & Cullum 1999)

research. This process is undertaken by many staff on diploma/degree/ENB courses and is the subject of many books in its own right. It is not therefore included here, but information is given in the Further reading section. This process has been done for you if there is a systematic review or a meta-analysis available.

MOVING TOWARDS EVIDENCE-BASED PRACTICE

Incorporating EBP into the perioperative environment involves a change in the way of thinking – the philosophy – of the department, as much as changes in particular practices.

The most fundamental part of this change of thinking is questioning practices going on around you. This does not need to be done in a challenging way but in a way that shows you are keen to find out more and get involved, whatever your clinical grade.

This way of thinking, of reviewing your practice and identifying problems, is part of a concept discussed elsewhere, that of being research minded. This is defined as follows: 'Being research minded means being aware of what literature is available and relevant to your area of work, and knowing how to read and implement it if appropriate' (Taylor 1998). Being research minded is therefore closely related to implementing EBP and can be seen as a precursor to developing EBP within a department. Box 10.3 shows ideas to consider in relation to being research minded and these are a useful move towards EBP.

Box 10.3   Are you research minded? (from Taylor 1998)

1. Do you question practices in your department or do you accept things as they are?
2. Do you recognise when a problem exists and act or ignore it?
3. Are the policies and procedures that underpin your work based on research or outdated rituals?
4. Are the policies and procedures in your department formulated by a multidisciplinary team who have used the available literature or are they put together by the chosen one or two, with no chance for discussion?
5. Do you read the relevant journals, so that you at least know what issues are under debate?
6. Do you read the supporting literature that accompanies new products, do you ask the rep for relevant research and read it with a questioning eye?
7. Do you ask your surgeons and anaesthetists for any relevant research for your department and ask them to explain it if you don't grasp it all?
8. Do you ask student nurses, ENB course nurses and student operating department practitioners if you can look at the work they are doing – case studies, projects, etc.?
9. Do you know where to find perioperative research or get help? Can you do a literature search?
10. Do you keep relevant articles for your speciality in your department?

Using evidence in practice – policies, procedures, standards, audit

Having accepted that incorporating evidence into your daily perioperative practice is a 'good thing', there are several steps involved before the evidence can be implemented. Once a literature search (by either traditional or electronic means) and a critical evaluation of the evidence have been completed, recommendations for practice within your own department should be evident. A vital part of EBP, and one that has received less attention in the journals, is putting it into practice – implementing the evidence.

Each department will have a variety of means to do this according to their structure and way of working. The theories of implementing change incorporate the features of getting agreement, getting people's involvement, cost analysis, giving information to others, supporting the staff and auditing the change in practice.

From a change management perspective, most changes in practice will have to go through the following steps.

- Presentation of the proposed change in practice to all staff involved with or affected by the change in practice.
- Agreement to the change from relevant department staff or nominated representatives, e.g. working group, policy committee, staff forum.

- Agreement to the change may also be needed from groups or individuals outside the operating department staff, such as occupational health, infection control or anaesthetic staff.
- The change in practice must be circulated to all staff and formally adopted from a particular date.

Wright (1998) provides further information on change, change strategies and acting as a change agent.

These points are all important in the event of any incident that may be related to the change in practice. The details of the change in practice, the date of its implementation and how staff were informed must be able to be demonstrated. This type of information should be held on record.

Exactly what form the change in practice will take will depend on what tools are used within the department – policies, procedures, clinical practices, standards or other audit tools. Each of these has advantages and disadvantages and operating department managers and staff should have identified which are the most appropriate for their department. A recommended change in practice can therefore be communicated to staff in the form of the new document (for example, policy or standard) with supporting evidence.

Tackling EBP in your department

As the previous sections have outlined, the implementation of EBP in the perioperative environment can be greatly enhanced by the concept of staff being research minded. This is therefore a useful starting place and some of the changes suggested in Box 10.3 are easy to implement.

More specific clinical practices can then be addressed and the impetus for these changes should arise from the review of your practice and identification of problems, as discussed earlier (p.163). A review of the working tools will identify the evidence in use, the policies, clinical practices, procedures or standards on which your work is based and all staff should be aware of this.

When beginning to implement EBP within the perioperative environment, a team of interested people is essential in order to share the workload and prevent the change in practice from being one person's project.

The team should then prioritise the problem areas identified and choose what appears to be the smallest topic for the first attempt at implementing EBP. A small change, possibly uniprofessional in nature, is possibly easier to tackle than bigger topics that require a multiprofessional, multidepartment approach. Unfortunately, most aspects of perioperative practice fit in the latter category! For example:

- discharge criteria for recovery units;
- frequency of observations/recording of observations in recovery units;
- length of scrubbing-up procedure;
- wearing of masks.

However, the main principle is that early projects should be as easy as possible, so that change can be implemented and results seen in practice.

Difficulties of utilisation

The difficulties of implementing research in clinical practice have been discussed and documented within nursing for many years. This problem remains even with the shift of emphasis towards the use of evidence and Newman et al (1998) identify barriers to implementing EBP as follows:

- Organisational
  - Low management priority
  - Difficulties with teamwork
  - Inadequate systems for managing personal and professional development
  - Difficulties in managing innovation
  - Inadequate systems for dissemination
  - Difficulties in accessing evidence
  - Resource constraints.
- Culture and practice of nursing
  - Motivation to change cannot be assumed
  - Ill-defined and competing interpretations of nursing roles and practice
  - Cultures emphasise 'doing' and inhibit questioning of practice (Newman et al 1998).

Many readers will recognise these barriers; they are similar to those discussed by Hunt (1981) many years ago and Carter more recently (1996) in relation to research. They can also be recognised in real life, in operating departments and other areas of health-care provision. They relate to difficulties in access to the evidence – how many staff are able to get to a library within their lunch break or even after work. Although this is the same for all areas of the hospital, the difficulty is compounded when additional time to change from theatre clothes is added to the equation. The barriers also relate to difficulties with the systems of work, the resources available and the people.

The people involved can be seen as key; as Newman et al (1998) discuss, 'Motivation to change practice cannot be assumed'. Ashworth (1998) supports this and identifies that clinical effectiveness in nursing can only be achieved if nurses are:

- well motivated;
- feeling valued and secure;
- well prepared in terms of basic and continuing education;
- well supported in terms of encouragement;
- well supported in terms of resources;
- given time for access and assessment of evidence;
- given time for planning, interaction and action to achieve change, and evaluation;

- able to use information technology or other necessary technical assistance;
- given management help to achieve organisational change to remove barriers to clinical effectiveness and other resources for effective practice.

Muir Gray (1997) supports this and highlights the key components of an evidence-based health service as both organisational and individual.

The difficulties of providing the work culture described above do not need to be highlighted to any member of operating department staff or their managers. The time and resources to implement EBP are difficult to achieve, given the service pressures we now live with. There are pressures on every surgeon and operating department to achieve waiting list targets and to complete waiting list initiatives.

These priorities of staff time to implement evidence-based clinically effective care and staff time to care for patients in order to prevent cancellations, are difficult ones to balance. All operating department staff must consider these two aspects of their role and consider, along with their managers, how they can be taken forward. Projects that identify how to implement change are therefore useful, even if the projects are not based within the perioperative environment: *Turning evidence into everyday practice* (PACE 1997), the interim report of the King's Fund PACE project, for example. This report shows that although change in practice can be achieved, it is a complex business. The PACE project has looked at the process of implementing clinical effectiveness across 16 UK sites, covering a range of clinical issues, e.g. pressure sore prevention and improving urinary continence. The final report is awaited at the time of publication.

CONCLUSION

This chapter has outlined both the concept and the practicality of EBP in the perioperative environment. It has aimed to provide the reader with an understanding of EBP and some ideas on how to move towards it. The amount of literature on this topic is vast and increasing daily as the knowledge base grows.

EBP is therefore a vital concept for perioperative staff. Cullum (1998) states that if we want an evidence-based health-care system, then evidence-based nursing is an essential component. On a national level it is apparent that we do want an evidence-based health-care system – it underpins both the Scottish and the English White Papers. It will not therefore go away!

It is a new area for most operating department staff and Smith (1997) provides a useful overview of EBP in the perioperative environment. This supports many of the concepts outlined within this chapter and in previous work (Taylor 1998). Not all nurses need to do research but they should be able to read and interpret research concerning their area of expertise and identify areas in which development or research is needed.

Cavanagh & Tross (1996) also state that nurses must be able to take their research knowledge base and create a protocol that is usable in the clinical area and to evaluate this. This, then, is the real use of EBP – something that can be used in practice to improve patient care.

Perioperative staff must therefore consider the ideas highlighted in this chapter and other literature and grasp the challenge and opportunity it presents each of us – to develop evidence-based practice in our own departments.

REFERENCES

Ashworth P 1998 Clinical effectiveness: an old ideal but with a newer context and approach in nursing (editorial). Intensive and Critical Care Nursing 14(4): 159–160

Ball J A 1989 Teaching materials. Quality Assurance Unit. Nuffield Institute for Health Service Studies, University of Leeds, Leeds

Carter D 1996 Barriers to the implementation of research findings in practice. Nurse Researcher 4(2): 30–40

Cavanagh S, Tross G 1996 Utilizing research findings in nursing: policy and practice considerations. Journal of Advanced Nursing 24(5): 1083–1088

Cullum N 1998 Evidence based practice. Nursing Management 5(3): 32–33

Culyer A 1995 Supporting research and development in the NHS. HMSO, London

Department of Health 1991 Research for health – a research and development strategy for the NHS. DoH, London

Fennessey G 1998 What's the evidence? Clinical effectiveness. RCN Nursing Update Learning Unit 087

Gray J 1997 Evidence based healthcare. Churchill Livingstone, Edinburgh

Heater B, Becker A, Olson R 1988 Nursing interventions and patient outcomes. A meta-analysis of studies. Nurse Researcher 37: 303–307

Hunt J 1981 Indicators for nursing practice: the use of research findings. Journal of Advanced Nursing 6(3): 189–194

Lewis B 1993 Diagnostic dilatation and curettage in young women. British Medical Journal 306(6872): 225–260

McMahon A 1997 Implications for nursing of the NHS R & D funding policy. Nursing Standard 28(11): 44–48

Morgan L, Fennessey G 1996 Levels of evidence. DQI Network News 4 3. Cited in McMahon A 1998 Developing practice through research. In: Roe B, Webb C (eds) Research and development in clinical nursing practice. Whurr, London

Muir Gray J 1997 Evidence based healthcare – how to make health policy and management decisions. Churchill Livingstone, New York

NATN 1998 Principles of safe practice in the perioperative environment. National Association of Theatre Nurses, Harrogate

NATN, AODP, BARNA, NHS Litigation Authority, MPS, RCN Perioperative Forum 1998 Safeguards for invasive procedures: the management of risks. National Association of Theatre Nurses, Harrogate

Newman M, Papadopoulos I, Sigsworth J 1998 Barriers to evidence based practice. Clinical Effectiveness in Nursing 2: 11–20

NHS Centre for Reviews and Dissemination 1996 Undertaking systematic reviews of research on effectiveness: CDR guidelines for those carrying out or commissioning reviews. NHS Centre for Reviews and Dissemination, York

NHSE 1996a Promoting clinical effectiveness – a framework for action in and through the NHS. NHSE, Leeds

NHSE 1996b Clinical guidelines – using clinical guidelines to improve patient care within the NHS. NHSE, Leeds

NHSE 1996c Clinical audit? Using clinical audit in the NHS: a position statement. NHSE, Leeds

Nursing and Midwifery Audit Service 1998 Levels of evidence: information for clinically effective practice. Information factsheet no. 3. NMAS, London

Nursing Standard and the Centre for Reviews and Dissemination 1997 Systematic reviews: examples for nursing. RCN Publishing, London

PACE Team 1997 Turning evidence into everyday practice. King's Fund, London

RCN 1990 Quality of patient care: the dynamic standard setting system. Scutari, Harrow

Sackett D, Haynes R, Guyatt G, Tugwell P 1991 Clinical epidemiology – a basic science for clinical medicine, 2nd edn. Little, Brown, Boston

Sackett D, Rosenberg W, Gray J, Hayes R, Richardson W 1996 Evidence based medicine: what it is and what it isn't. British Medical Journal 312: 71–72

Smith C 1997 Evidence based nursing. Nursing Management 3(10): 22–23

Taylor M 1998 Are you research minded? British Journal of Theatre Nursing 7(12): 27–30

Thompson C, Cullum N 1999 Examining evidence: an overview. Nursing Times Learning Curve 3(1): 7–9

Thompson D 1998 Why evidence based nursing? Nursing Standard 13(9): 58–59

Walsh M 1998 Evidence based practice: is patient satisfaction evidence? Nursing Standard 12(49): 38–42

Walsh M, Ford P 1989 Nursing rituals – research and rational actions. Heinemann, Oxford

Wicker P 1997 Sacred cows and sound practice. British Journal of Theatre Nursing 7(7): 31–34

Wright S 1998 Changing nursing practice, 2nd edn. Arnold, London

---

FURTHER READING AND INFORMATION

Searching the literature

Connell D 1998 Learning to retrieve. Nursing Times Learning Curve 1(11): 4–6

McKibbon K, Marks S 1998 Searching for the best evidence. Part 2 Searching CINAHL and Medline. Evidence-Based Nursing 1(4): 105–107

Reading the evidence

Smith P (ed) 1997 Research mindedness for practice – an interactive approach for nursing and health care. Churchill Livingstone, New York

Hendry C, Farley A 1988 Reviewing the literature: a guide for students. Nursing Standard 12(44): 46–48

Evidence-based practice – general

Kitson A 1997 Using evidence to demonstrate the value of nursing. Nursing Standard 11(28): 34–39

RCN/RCM clinical audit information service bibliography series:
No. 9 – Guidelines, protocols, criteria and standards
No. 10 – Evidence based practice and clinical effectiveness

Nursing and midwifery audit information service factsheets:
No. 3 – Levels of evidence. Information for clinically effective practice

CINAHL – an index of health-care journals on CD-ROM in most nursing/medical libraries. Emphasis is on nursing.

Medline – an electronic version of the Index Medicus, on CD-ROM in most nursing/medical libraries.

USEFUL ADDRESSES

Centre for Evidence-Based Nursing
Department of Health Studies
University of York
Genesis 6
York Science Park
York YO10 5DQ

UK Cochrane Centre
NHS R & D Programme
Summertown Pavilion
Middleway
Oxford OX2 7LG

NHS Centre for Reviews and Dissemination
University of York
Heslington
York YO1 5DD

RCN Institute Dynamic Quality Improvement Programme
20 Cavendish Square
London W1M 0AB

RCN Nursing and Midwifery Audit Information Service
20 Cavendish Square
London W1M 0AB

SIGN – Scottish Intercollegiate Network
Administration Support Group
Royal College of Physicians
9 Queen Street
Edinburgh EH2 1JQ

St George's Health Care Evaluation Unit
Blackshaw Road
Tooting
London SW17 0QT

PACE
King's Fund Development Centre
11–13 Cavendish Square
London W1M 0AN

GRIPP (Getting Research into Purchasing and Practice)
Project Manager
Anglia and Oxford Regional Office
Old Road
Headington
Oxford OX3 7LF

Website addresses

Evidence-Based Nursing journal
    http://www.evidencebasdnursing.com

Cochrane Centre
    http://hiru.mcmaster.ca/cochrane/

NHS Centre for Reviews and Dissemination
http://york.ac.uk/inst/crd

Bandolier – a monthly newsletter summarising reviews and reports of effectiveness
http://www/jr2.ox.ac.uk/Bandolier

Budgeting

Kate Woodhead

This chapter describes the broad issues in public health finances, the recent changes (some of which are not yet in place), and where possible links the broad picture to the financial issues in perioperative care delivery. In order to understand how funding for the NHS works, it is necessary to look at where the money comes from and to follow it through it's course. The principles inherent in funding healthcare discussed below refer to the United Kingdom prior to devolution. This may in future result in differing perspectives, but the principles ought to remain the same.

THE BIG PICTURE

In the year 1998–9 the total NHS budget was £37.2 billion in England, Scotland and Wales, which is equivalent to £103 million per day. This was increased by the Labour government, in a major review of public spending, on a 3-year basis to a target of £46 billion in 2001–2. This is an innovation in public spending and aims to move from the hitherto customary annual spending round to place plans for public expenditure on a more stable 3-year basis (NHS Budget, *The Times* July 15 1998).

Funding for the NHS has been based in the past on a competitive internal market set up by the reforms of the previous government. The White Paper *The new NHS: modern, dependable* (DoH 1997) proposes that the internal market be replaced by a more collaborative system of 'integrated care' based on 'partnership' and driven by 'performance' (Goddard & Mannion 1998).

The cost of providing NHS health care in 1998–9 was £37.2 billion which was approximately 11% of total public spending in that period. Eighty-three percent of NHS finance is provided through general taxation, a further 13% comes from the NHS element of National Insurance contributions while most of the remainder (4%) is accounted for by user charges, such as prescription charges and dental care.

Although most comparable countries also rely overwhelmingly on public finance to fund their health-care systems, the United Kingdom is unusual in the extent to which it depends upon general taxation as a source of funding (NAHAT 1994).

The finance initiatives described below refer to the White Papers published in England and Wales and in Scotland. Changes in Northern Ireland where a Green Paper was published (DoH 1998), are still subject to consultation.

The UK system for the allocation of resources to different regions of the country is to change as part of the White Paper. Essentially the pie will be divided by central government using a 'needs based' formula. The current system is a formula using weighted capitation where crude population data are weighted by age, need and market force factors (Miller 1998).

In the future, local health authorities will be informed of their allocation of money by central government. This will then be divided amongst a number of locality-based commissioning groups. These primary care groups replaced general practitioner fund-holding practices in April 1999 and will bring together GPs and community nurses in a given area who will be responsible for commissioning services for the local community. Primary care groups will serve populations of 100 000. They will hold a single budget in order to purchase health care for their population.

Health authorities meanwhile will develop a 3-year health improvement programme (HIP) to identify local health needs. The primary care groups must spend their money in a way that is consistent with the local HIP. The HIP will decide the range of services needed for the local population (DoH 1997). The details of how primary care groups are to function are not yet clear, but it is implied in the White Paper that the groups will commission contracts for care with acute trusts, social services and local community services on a 3-year basis. Trusts will continue to be responsible for operational management and will also be involved in drawing up the local HIP. Trusts will have combined quality and financial duties for the first time (DoH 1997).

Finance for providers

The terms 'purchaser' and 'provider' are no longer used to denote health authorities and GP fund holders who used to contract with hospitals for care. The White Paper describes a 'third' way which maintains the separation between 'planning' and 'provision'.

One of the new ways in which the new collaborative partnerships are to be forged is via the replacement of the annual contracting round with longer term funding agreements for the provision of health-care services covering periods of 3–5 years (DoH 1997). Within this new framework of integrated care, the longer term agreements are seen as developing a more cooperative service and a way of allowing clinicians and managers to focus on improving care. Sharing information between the planners and the providers will be key in the new cooperation and partnership arrangements and will be based on trust.

Income and expenditure

Contracts for provision of services will be based on the needs of the local population and will be commissioned by the primary care groups. Acute hospital trusts will be in a position to focus on delivering care according to

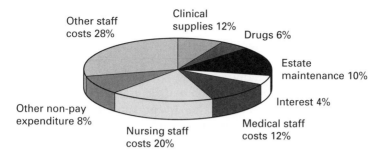

Figure 11.1   Trust expenditure

the local HIP (which they will have helped to develop) on a more stable basis as the plans will be in place for 3–5 years.

The golden rule which was applied to all NHS trusts by the health reforms of the 1990s is that expenditure must not exceed income. As described above, the cash limits within public sector spending will not alter with the changes implicit in the White Paper and all trusts must stay within budget.

Trusts will be responsible, as they are now, for the internal allocation of budgets. A typical trust budget might divide income for any given year into the divisions shown in Figure 11.1, in the expectation that expenditure will fall into approximately these percentages.

Capital and revenue

Capital assets are best defined as those that are substantial and durable and are used by an organisation over a number of years: for example, land, plant and equipment. Revenue expenditure, in contrast, is the finance needed to run the organisation on a day-to-day basis. These include pay, consumables and small items of equipment.

In the NHS there are special terms which define capital assets. Capital assets are single items with an expected life of more than a year and with a value of more than £5000. Some collective assets may also come into this definition, provided that they are collectively worth more than £5000 and they are bought together, used together and disposed of at the same time.

Budgeting is part of a financial cycle that aims to plan and control agreed activities and is the financial target that must be met if we are to live within our means. The business planning cycle includes service and activity planning, service contracting and human resource planning as well as the annual budget-setting process.

Budget-setting process

The budget for different hospital departments usually concerns only the day-to-day expenditure, i.e. revenue monies. The budget-setting process is likely to begin with a draft proposal from the accountants (usually based largely on last year's spending patterns), taking particular cost pressures, which have been identified within the hospital or department, into consideration.

The draft budget is usually available by the beginning of the financial year, but currently is entirely dependent on the contract prices with all major purchasers being agreed. The 3-year contracts suggested by the White Paper ensure that a far more streamlined approach to annual budget setting is possible as the income will be more stable year on year. Revision of the draft budget takes place when prices have been agreed and the full income for the financial year can be assessed.

The cake can then be cut into the appropriate number of slices. The operating department may be divided into speciality sections or may be a whole-department budget. In the author's experience, the smaller the slice, the easier it is to trace and monitor expenditure closely.

Budgeting is thus an ongoing process throughout the financial year (usually April 1 to March 31) to monitor the monthly expenditure against the monthly target.

Annual report and accounts

As with any business, trusts have to be accountable to the public and to the NHS Executive for use of their financial resources. Each year, a set of accounts is published as an income and expenditure account, a balance sheet and a cash flow statement. These statements have to be audited by the Audit Commission, an independent body appointed by the government (the Accounts Commission in Scotland) to give a true and fair view of each trust's performance.

Income and expenditure account

This shows the income earned from patient contracts and other sources, how much has been spent to achieve the income and the record of the surplus or loss incurred.

Balance sheet

A balance sheet is a picture – a freeze frame – of a trust's finances at a particular moment in time. It is called a balance sheet as it is a measure of the money flowing into and out of a closed system. The money flowing 'in' must equal the money flowing 'out'.

Cash flow statement

This shows the flows of cash both into and out of the trust from all sources. It may also be known as the liquidity position statement.

Annual statements are published of the state of a trust's activities during the previous financial year and will be included in its audited accounts. This is usually in the form of a glossy brochure, published to coincide with the annual general meeting.

OPERATING DEPARTMENT BUDGETS

Types of budget

There are various approaches to preparing a budget that may be used by a hospital. The commonest types in use in the NHS are:

- incremental budgeting;
- zero-based budgets;
- activity-based budgets;

each of which will be briefly described.

Incremental budgeting

This uses the current year's budget as a base for setting the following year's and is the simplest to use and understand. Fortunately, it is commonly used in health care and is undemanding on accountants' and budget holder's time. It is based on history with some adjustments made for several factors.

- *Non-recurring items*, which may be a sum for an agreed number of speciality patients on a waiting list initiative.
- *Full year effects*, which might be a new post created halfway through the year which will have to be made up to account for the full year salary next year.
- *Changes in service*, which might be a new session created according to a change in the contract for a speciality.
- *Cost improvement programme*, that is, a target set by government to deliver efficiency savings. Hospitals have a number of ways of delivering these, the most usual being to ask each budget holder to have a certain percentage less on their budget annually so that this is spread evenly across all areas of the hospital. It is commonly known as a CIP and is widely used in this abbreviated form.

Zero-based budgeting

This is a technique which assumes that budgets start from scratch each year with specification of the quality and quantity of activity to be delivered, looking at optimum numbers of staff, equipment, accommodation and consumables to deliver the contracted service requirement. Essentially, this involves an annual challenge to the cost of service delivery and can for that reason be a very effective way of managing change and challenging assumptions. However, it is very costly to operate, as the process annually is a lengthy one and may be time wasting.

Activity-based budgeting

The fixed (pay) and variable (consumables and overtime, etc.) elements of the budget are set separately. This budget type allows flexibility of the budget when activity (which affects the variable element) varies from the plan. This type of budget is well suited to operating department budgets and would be used more widely if the information systems to supply activity data were more sophisticated than they generally are.

Balancing the budget

Those responsible for spending taxpayer's money are repeatedly urged to 'get more for less'. This certainly applies in health care and is the maxim used to ensure that efficiency, value for money and cost-effective care are at the top of the public sector agenda.

It is helpful to imagine that the budget-balancing activity that must go on month on month in an operating department is no different, other than in scale, from managing one's domestic budget. The income, i.e. pay cheque each month, is the sum against which all the household bills, petrol, holidays and fun have to be metered out. Each month there will be similar amounts of expenditure for regular fixed costs, e.g. debits for insurance, local taxes and the mortgage, and in addition there are varied amounts each month for petrol, food and fun. One has to keep some in reserve for one-off payments for the car service, television licence or holiday costs. The costs of all of these must be no greater than the monthly salary or the budget will not balance at the end of the month.

Close monitoring of all the costs associated with an operating department budget, or a part of the whole, to meet the monthly targets is an important element of managing any budget. If possible, some funds should be kept in reserve for large bills such as the annual maintenance cost for the microscopes or equivalent.

Activity levels are not usually within the control of the budget holder but the constant requirement to stay within the budget must be at the top of every user's mind so that waste and unnecessary costs are kept to a minimum and control of expenditure is maintained.

Reporting mechanisms

These will vary to some extent but, commonly, a report is provided by the hospital accountants to record expenditure for specific budget holders, listing pay and non-pay items purchased during the course of a month or there may be more sophisticated reports which show the balance of income and expenditure to a budget code.

It is clearly the responsibility of budget holders to read and understand these reports so that they will recognise any peaks and troughs of spending and can keep mental notes of where there has to be 'less' next month and where there is room for manoeuvre, perhaps to allow purchase of 'one-off' items, next month. The accountant is on hand to explain and clarify the reports with the budget holder. It is useful to have a regular monthly review of the reports with the accountant.

Fixed and variable costs

These are commonly used terms to describe elements of the budget. Fixed costs are those that do not vary according to activity, e.g. most of the pay budget is a fixed cost.

Variable costs are those that do vary month to month, e.g. the enhanced hours for weekend and evening work will vary according to the level of pay of each worker and the number of hours those staff worked. Consumables and drugs in an operating department budget are variable costs according to the level of activity and these will change month by month.

Capital expenditure

Capital assets are best defined as those that are substantial and durable and are used by an organisation over a number of years, e.g. land, plant and equipment. Revenue expenditure, in contrast, is the finance needed to run the organisation on a day-to-day basis; for example, pay, consumables and small items of equipment.

Allocation of capital monies is organised in different ways in different hospitals but the most common practice is an annual set of bids which are prioritised by management. Operating departments usually have a high quantity of capital items which need regular replacement. If the hospital requires a prioritised list to be produced, it is usually necessary to put this together as a business case or a slightly less formal 'case of need'.

Most bids for a new capital item will have some revenue consequences. For example, a bid for a new diathermy machine will need to include regular maintenance and disposable items in order to make it useable for patients. Estimates or quotations for revenue consequences are usually required as part of the purchasing process.

Capital charges were introduced to the NHS in 1991 and are the method by which an organisation spreads the cost of acquiring capital assets over the lifetime of the assets themselves. This can be likened to being charged a hire cost for the use of the assets; the current charge levied by the Department of Health on individual hospitals is 6% on all capital assets. This demonstrates the importance of holding an accurate and up-to-date asset register of all major equipment assets held by the hospital.

Each business case written to demonstrate the need for a new piece of equipment should have financial information included which details the net cash flow, net present value, capital charges and revenue consequences. This is organised according to accounting techniques by the supporting accountant for the operating department and should demonstrate a process called 'whole life costing'.

During the business planning cycle, it is common for operating departments to review their equipment needs for the year ahead and to identify replacement items. However, trusts with severe cost pressures have considerably reduced capital available annually for replacement items, which may mean waiting for a piece of equipment to break down irrevocably before the process to find capital funds to replace it is started.

Cases of need

Many hospitals, departments or managers will ask for 'cases of need' to be produced to exert some control over the purchase of new equipment. For the purposes of understanding it does not matter whether the item is a new and costly instrument or a type of consumable which has not previously been bought by the department. This is an excellent way of learning the formal process of writing a full business case for a new capital item. The case of need could include the following headings.

- Current provision.
- Background, if it is to support a service development.
- What will the capital cost be (attach quotation)?
- Does this include the negotiated price or is it list price?
- Are there revenue consequences? What are they (attach quotation)?
- What is the consequence to the service if this item is not purchased?

The supplies department and accountant should be aware of the submission of a case of need as they can help with the negotiation of the best offer from the company and understand how much you need the item(s). They will also help prepare the financial information in an appropriate form for the hospital.

COST EFFECTIVENESS IN PERIOPERATIVE CARE

Pressure on cost effectiveness in operating departments has never been greater and the emphasis is on delivering an efficient service with close monitoring of all expenditure that occurs. Managers are increasingly required to account for the costs of their services and, in varying detail, to justify all expenditure.

Staffing costs

Pay budgets in the operating department are likely to represent as much as 70% of the total cost of providing the service. It is for this reason that pressure is often focused in this area and in times of financial crisis, the hospital's response may be to impose a vacancy freeze. A higher percentage of costs can be saved quickly by not filling vacancies as the fixed cost element of the budget will show savings immediately.

However, recruitment of new staff can be a lengthy and frustrating business when, as now, there is a shortage of appropriately qualified staff available in the market place. Given that there is a chronic shortage of perioperative staff available to recruit, vacancies may well take some time to fill and thus the 'savings' required will be achieved before an appropriate appointment is made. In the author's experience, when there are vacancies in operating departments, the department's response is to increase the overtime available for existing staff (variable cost element in the budget) in order to provide a service to patients. This is a far more costly option, in more than just financial terms, than employing new staff to fill vacancies.

Establishment

The term used to identify the numbers of staff required to run an operating department service and set up the appropriate budget to pay them is 'establishment'. How does one set up an establishment to reflect accurately the numbers of staff required and at which grades? The National Association of Theatre Nurses (NATN) is often asked for guidance on the numbers of staff required to deliver the service. This is never clearcut and although a guide to establishing staffing numbers has been published (NATN 1995), local conditions should always be applied to any staffing needs assessment.

It is important to assess the activity and department profile in order to identify the numbers and grades of staff required. Skill mix appropriate to the complexity of service or throughput of patients is also an important consideration.

Sickness and absence management

Absence management has been particularly highlighted in hospitals recently since government policy changed to employers bearing the costs of staff absence. Sickness policies for management of short-term and intermittent absence as well as the management of long-term sickness have been in greater evidence as the real cost of time off sick is increasingly counted. The national average is quoted as 4% and hospitals and in particular operating departments appear to have higher than the national average levels of sickness.

The cost to teams and individuals of continuing sickness is high in financial terms, particularly if the absence has to be paid for twice by employing agency staff or the use of overtime to enable uninterrupted service delivery to patients.

Detailed analysis and management of sickness is therefore implicit in delivering a cost-effective service. The ideal culture in an operating department is one where individuals feel that attendance is important. The other principle which should be demonstrable is that individuals are treated fairly and consistently. An active approach to management of sickness should encourage staff to feel valued and highlight their individual contribution to service delivery.

Utilisation and planning of services

Most operating departments work to a weekly session schedule, unlike the private sector where the emphasis may have to be more flexible. The major costs are those of staffing a session and it is therefore imperative that an operating department can demonstrate that staff costs are optimised by matching work load to staff rosters. Audits of the value for money of operating departments focus on shift times, unused sessions and staff redeployment. Whilst it is recognised that there are 'other' responsibilities and duties involved in delivering a service in an operating department, it should also be possible to regularly analyse and report on session utilisation.

Operating department management systems or hospital information systems can produce reports to describe utilisation that is usually expressed as a percentage of available time. If this is undertaken manually the method used is to divide the number of hours actually used by the number of elective hours available and staffed and then this is expressed as a percentage. The Bevan Report (NHS Management Executive 1989) described a target of 90% as the ideal utilisation for operating departments.

Planning for new services

Maximising income opportunities by developing new services, waiting list initiatives and reduction of underutilised sessions, perhaps by replacing them with a different speciality list, are frequent planning needs in an operating department. Assessing the needs of a service includes estimations of effective skill mix for the perioperative service, portering requirements and details of budget changes implied by the change of service. Staffing costs as well as other service delivery costs, such as laundry, CSSD and consumables, should be included in any assessment for the costs of providing a new session or service.

Documentation of the changes proposed and the method by which the new service was estimated is helpful later, if one needs to demonstrate that the estimate was insufficient to deliver the service effectively and efficiently. It is always useful to have a historical trace on how the establishment changes have occurred.

Monitoring systems

Operating department management systems have revolutionised the ability of an operating department to analyse cost-effective service delivery. They are able to deliver regular reports on activity, session utilisation and the variance between staff hours planned and actual hours used, amongst other things. The complexity of modern operating department service delivery and the increasing need by hospitals to demonstrate value for money mean that they must be produced manually in the absence of computerisation.

Control of expenditure is difficult without regular reports and managers may be under special pressure to deliver them on a regular basis. This in turn has implications for all staff who have responsibility for documentation, rostering and out-of-hours planning of staff. Requests for information that is accurate and timely are increasing, in order to analyse the service delivery and control expenditure.

Information regularly required on perioperative service delivery may include some or all of the following (or more!).

- Sickness, annual leave and study leave by employee.
- Establishment details with vacancies or overestablishment highlighted.
- Activity levels according to corporate data needs, usually speciality based.

- Activity recorded by elective and acute (emergency) cases.
- Utilisation percentage may be by speciality. Underruns/overruns by consultant.
- Private patient activity.
- Reasons for cancellation of sessions and patients.

It is extremely time consuming to collect these data, organise and present them regularly but it is necessary in our pressured financial climate. It may be worth considering the employment of a clerical officer with spread-sheet skills within an operating department to deliver these regularly or, at a far higher cost, implement a theatre management system. The Bevan Report (NHS Management Executive 1989) highlights the need for operating departments to invest in information systems to deliver the data required.

Materials management

The management of stocks and supplies in operating departments is a costly and complex business. Streamlining the supply chain (the chain of events used to describe the process from ordering an item to its final delivery) to reduce costs to the department and hospital is a very effective method of demonstrating continuing downward pressure on procedure costs.

The essence of materials management is to ensure that an optimum number of individual items are available as required for patients, without compromising a quality service. The objective is to manage products in such a way that overall stock holding is reduced and replenished as necessary, rather than having products on the shelf 'just in case' they are required. Duplication of stock should be avoided as much as possible and items need to be rotated on the shelf to ensure they remain in date.

It is possible to manage 'just-in-time' supplies to operating theatres providing that deliveries are frequent. Logistics companies are developing business arrangements with health-care organisations to provide back-up products of a specified range which can be supplied and delivered 'just in time'. New ways to procure supplies are being explored all the time and can represent huge savings for hospitals, but may require new ways of working and development of trusting partnerships with suppliers.

There are now a variety of procedure packs available to reduce shelf stocks of frequently used combinations of products. Assessment of the core contents of the procedure packs is essential, as is supplies support for negotiating a good pricing system for the procedure packs. Valuable professional time can be saved by using these packs, where procedures are likely to be relatively standard in a speciality or where the consultant's surgical practice is consistent and predictable.

Professional time spent ordering supplies should be delegated to support staff who may be theatre support workers, supplies staff or specially trained materials management staff. Control of initial item selection and stock levels should be retained by perioperative staff.

Rationalisation of products

Challenges should regularly be made by all perioperative staff to the items they are using in order to justify them. Standardisation of products such as catheters and dressings will save money on 'high-volume, low-cost' items whilst reduction in the range of stapling devices or orthopaedic prostheses will save on 'high-cost, low volume' items. The decisions should be made in full consultation with clinicians and all potential users. Supplies department staff should also be involved as they fully understand the nature of changing products and can ensure best practice in pricing, delivery and contract negotiation.

Costs of individual consumables should be known by perioperative staff, although it is recognised that this is time consuming to keep 'live' and up to date. Operating departments are constantly bombarded with new products. Surgical techniques develop very quickly and it is easy to consume the budget if new items are not carefully screened for their cost effectiveness. It is essential to ensure that individual products are not purchased without a full understanding of what they will replace and the cost of purchase. Contracts and prices should be negotiated by supplies staff with estimates of annual use to ensure the best prices.

CONCLUSION

Operating department costs continue to rise with advancing technology and with much of the pressure in health care focused on balancing of budgets, there will never again be a time when cost pressures are not keenly felt by those working in the perioperative environment. It is essential that those working and managing within this area are well educated and understand the analysis required on a regular basis to trace and account for expenditure. Downward pressure on unit costs is essential in all areas of business and an operating department is a specific hospital area which must continue to show close monitoring, analysis and reduction of costs in any area possible. Those responsible for delivery of the service are required to be constantly looking for new ways to deliver a value-for-money service so it is necessary to understand how the money is currently allocated and spent.

REFERENCES

Department of Health 1997 The new NHS: modern, dependable. The Stationery Office, London.
Department of Health 1998 Designed to care. Renewing the NHS in Scotland. The Stationery Office, London
Goddard M, Mannion R 1998 From competition to co-operation: new economic relationships in the National Health Service. Health Economics 7(2): 105–119
Miller P 1998 Adding to local divisions. Health Service Journal 108(5590): 28–29
NAHAT 1994 Health and the economy. Research paper 14. National Association of Health Authorities and Trusts, Birmingham

NATN 1995 Staffing in the operating department. National Association of Theatre Nurses, Harrogate
NHS Management Executive 1989 The Bevan Report. HMSO, London

FURTHER READING

Audit Commission 1996 Goods for your health. Audit Commission Publications, London
Harrison J 1989 Finance for the non-financial manager. Thorsons, London

Information technology

Paul Wicker

COMPUTER DEVELOPMENT

The history of computer development is short but explosive. The first IBM personal computer came onto the market about 20 years ago and these early computers, for example, the Intel 4004, although a masterpiece for its time, could only process four items of information at once. Entry-level Pentium computers are now infinitely more powerful and many can boast 15 gigabyte (Gb) hard disks, 128 MB memory and 600 MHz chips.

IBM, at that time the most influential computer manufacturer, needed a 'user-friendly' language for its computers so it asked Microsoft to produce an operating system, which it called 'DOS'. This quickly developed into 'Windows' and the rest is history. Computers have become more appealing to the public, largely because of the popularity of Windows 3.x and now Windows 95 and the Web-enhanced Windows 98. This has ensured that the personal computer has had an impact on practically every home and office in the country.

The latest and most exciting development has been the Internet, which has become accessible to more people as cheaper and faster modems have developed.

UNDERSTANDING COMPUTERS

A computer is, very basically, composed of three main parts:

1. the central processing unit (CPU);
2. the random access memory (RAM);
3. the storage medium (normally the hard drive).

The 'motherboard' links all the components of the computer by an incredibly complicated network of electrical pathways. Other components of the computer system include the video screen, which is required in order to see 'what is going on', and the keyboard and mouse which input commands or information into the computer. There is also a huge variety of 'add-ons', such as tape drives, scanners, CD-ROMs and video cameras.

Box 12.1   Computer components

RAM (random access memory) – the more RAM a computer has, the more programs it can run. RAM is electronic memory which is stored in RAM chips (integrated circuits) called SIMMS (single in-line memory modules). The information contained in these RAM chips is lost whenever the computer is turned off.

CD-ROM drive – a CD-ROM is a disk which contains information etched into it. Each disk can hold about 650 Mb of memory. Its main uses include storage of large quantities of information for databases or for multimedia uses (sound, video clips, pictures, etc.).

Floppy disk drive – the advantage of the floppy disk drive over the hard disk drive is that it enables information to be physically transported between computers.

Hard disk drive – this is used to store a computer's data and programs and acts as the computer's filing cabinet.

ROM (read only memory) – instructions in the ROM drive basic programs that activate and prepare the computer for use with an operating system such as DOS.

CPU (central processing unit) – this 'chip' is responsible for processing information or instructions and carrying out the user's commands. The CPU's speed of operation is measured in MHz (the latest Pentiums currently run at 600 MHz).

Motherboard – the motherboard is probably the most important part of the computer because it is a major factor in the overall speed of the computer.

Expansion board – these are used to connect peripherals such as scanners and video cards to the computer.

Video screen – this allows the user to see the effect of inputting information into the computer.

Keyboard – this is the main information input device for the computer.

Pointing device – these include devices such as the mouse, light pens and graphic tablets.

APPLICATIONS PACKAGES

A computer performs a specific series of tasks, including the following.
- Common applications
    Word processing
    Spreadsheets
    Databases
    Desktop publishing
    Graphics packages

- Specialised applications
    Catalogues
    Operating room information systems
- Educational applications
    Encyclopaedias
    Edutainment
    Interactive databases
    Training programs

COMMON APPLICATIONS

Word processing

Word processors extend the functions of an electronic typewriter to an incredible extent. Programs that perform these tasks include Word for Windows, WordPerfect for Windows and Lotus Ami Pro.

There are two basic advantages of word processors over typewriters. A word processor saves information so that it only has to be typed once and can be easily adapted for a number of different purposes. Also, word processors allow easy editing of written words without having to retype everything. Beyond this, they can perform miracles such as electronically cutting and pasting text from one article to another, inserting graphics such as pictures, boxes and frames and indexing or sorting text.

Spreadsheets

Spreadsheets are applications that can perform calculations and manipulate numerical data such as graphs and tables. Examples include Excel, Lotus 1-2-3 for Windows and Quattro Pro for Windows. A spreadsheet can perform complex functions and statistical analysis as well as performing basic sums (for example, adding, subtracting and dividing). A spreadsheet could, for example, collate data, analyse percentages and other statistics and produce a table and chart of the results. The main advantage of spreadsheets over manual calculations is that they can work very quickly. They also have a huge storage potential and they can automatically recalculate the whole table of results if part of the original data changes.

Databases

Databases are collections of information – anything from address books to surgeon's preference cards, diaries and accounting systems. Retrieval of information is easy because items of information are ordered and indexed. Programs that can do this include dBase, Paradox and Access. Linking the information to other programs (such as a word processor) can help to produce names and addresses or reports. One of the advantages of using databases is the ease with which information can be sorted and filtered.

This can be a huge advantage when the database contains large amounts of information, such as in an address book.

Desktop publishing (DTP)

A word processor provides an easy way of getting words onto paper, with the secondary intent of making it look professional and pleasing to the eye. A desktop publisher looks at the problem the other way around – it looks first at the layout on paper and it adds text and other items later.

DTP replaces traditional typesetting for the production of most modern published work. The program places text and graphics on a page and these objects can then be rotated, cropped or manipulated to produce the final layout. Popular programs include Aldus PageMaker, Quark Xpress and Serif's PagePlus.

Graphics

These programs make or manipulate pictures that are stored, displayed or printed.

Paint programs, such as Picture Publisher and Corel Photopaint, can perform extremely intricate and astounding changes to photos. They have tools that can, for example, change the contrast, brightness or colours in photos, very much like a conventional darkroom. Special effects, such as 'emboss', 'smear' and 'oil paint', can be used to change the appearance of the photo completely.

Vector programs are useful for producing images such as line drawings or relatively simple 'cartoons'. These programs simply recalculate the equations related to line lengths, curves and angles of a picture to increase or decrease pictures to any size. They are very useful for producing shapes that need to be resized without losing any of their resolution or sharpness (for example, company logos).

SPECIALISED APPLICATIONS

Catalogues

Online catalogues are popular for a number of reasons. First they can be searched easily because they are electronically based. Searching can be by key word, product reference, product name and so on. The second point is that online catalogues are very compact as they can be stored on CD-ROM. It is quite possible for an entire company's product range to be stored on one CD-ROM. The more sophisticated online catalogues can link to faxes or email and automatically generate requisition forms which can be sent directly to the company's sales points.

Ethicon have produced a very slick selection of catalogues for its various companies, with Ethicon Endosurgery's catalogue being a prime example. These catalogues are on the WorldWide Web and can be found at:

www.ethicon.com/wound_management/product/index.htm and www.ethicon-endo.com/

Ethicon Endosurgery's catalogue lists various products including stapling and ligation, videoscopic and Ultracision products. Using buttons, the user can undertake a catalogue search by inputting various key words and be rewarded with information such as product numbers, specifications and even full colour photographs.

Howmedica's catalogue is also available on the WorldWide Web at: www.howmedica.com

This catalogue boasts an extremely user-friendly interface and some useful additions in the form of explanations to surgical procedures and clinical trial results.

Information systems

Various information systems have been developed over the last few years that enable theatre management to improve the efficiency of their operating departments. One of the most popular systems is ORSOS.

The ORSOS theatre management system is a comprehensive surgical information system which brings together all the different elements of resource management including case scheduling, staff scheduling, equipment maintenance, inventory control, patient charting and management reporting. Its purpose is to increase the efficiency of a department and bring about improved cost control. The original ORSOS was a DOS-based program but the latest incarnation, ORSOS 3, is a Windows 95 product which has all the advantages of a user-friendly and intuitive interface. The four main modules include case scheduling, resource database, inventory control and management reporting.

The case-scheduling module automates the appointment books across all surgical specialities and manipulates information which has been input from the operating rooms. This enables the recording of 'real-time' case activities, printing of schedules, recording cases and providing daily reports such as intraoperative data records, daily statistics, admission reports and daily assignment worksheets.

The resource database is a record of resources available to the theatre management: for example, staff members, suites and sessions available, surgical equipment and instrument trays. These resources can be monitored and also procedures such as preventive maintenance schedules can be linked to the information.

The inventory control module provides warehouse inventory control which can be linked to surgeons' preference cards. This enables the fast and direct monitoring of the anticipated and actual use of resources for each case. Costing or charging information is also integrated into this module and can be sent to finance centres. Management reports can be generated and used for controlling and reducing inventory cost. Such reports include purchase orders, implant records, inventory usage, cost per procedure and stock reports.

The management reporting schedule module reports on the department's work practices. Reports include number of patients, operating theatre utilisation, productivity, procedure costs, time per procedure, cancellation reports and so on. The information can be represented in tabular or graph form for easy interpretation.

Various expansion modules can be added to the basic ORSOS 3 system: for example, personnel scheduling, which is an automated 'off duty' rostering system, and perioperative charting which is a sophisticated charting system which can monitor the patient throughout the length of their treatment in the hospital.

EDUCATION PACKAGES

Computers use a whole range of media (such as video, pictures, sound, text and animation) to impart information. This enhances the learning experience in a variety of ways.

Encyclopaedias

Three of the most popular electronic encyclopaedias are *Encarta*, *Encyclopaedia Britannica* and *Hutchinson's Encyclopaedia*. *Encarta*, which has now become a standard item for most PC users, combines many features that other programs have also adopted. The user can, for example, search for an article by keyword, browse through associated topics, electronically cut and paste text or pictures from the program to their article. The article can then be printed out with automatic referencing in order to have a permanent record or to provide handouts. These encyclopaedias can also integrate many other features, such as word searching, complex subject searches, interactive quizzes, automatic updating of the information through the Internet or interactive lectures.

Edutainment

The stimulating way of presenting information on screen has generated huge interest. Edutainment is a 'fun' or interesting way of learning. Normally these packages focus on a particular subject and aim to provide the user with general information. Examples include Dorling Kindersley's *Ultimate human skeleton* and Guildsoft's *BodyWorks*.

Interactive databases

A CD-ROM database can store over 65 million words. This vast amount of information can be easily retrieved and manipulated. This has led to the production of vast databases that are easily available to the general public.

Epic, for example, has produced a CD-ROM that includes information from the (anonymous) medical records of over 6 million people, gleaned from the General Practice Research Database. This information is updated every 6 months. Using this database, researchers can analyse the numbers of patients in the UK with certain diseases, symptoms, conditions and medical and surgical interventions. Each area of interest can be further split by factors such as patients' age, sex and geographic location.

Multimedia training programs

The most useful aspect of these programs is the ability to combine the various elements of media to involve the user in the learning process. For example, the user can interact with the program to carry out activities. There is also an element of being able to manipulate the program and influence the way it progresses. This is true interactivity that would be impossible with a video-based training programme.

Several organisations are now developing training packages. For example, Ethicon has produced an interactive tutorial on the use of sutures. Valleylab UK is currently producing an interactive tutorial on the process of tissue density feedback, a technology associated with electrosurgery. This program takes the user through a short educational session (using the analogy of a book) and then finishes off with a self-assessment questionnaire. The National Association of Theatre Nurses has produced a multimedia edition of the book *Working with electrosurgery*.

THE INFLUENCE OF THE INTERNET

The Internet began its life in the United States as a government program designed to defend its computer systems against nuclear attack by a communist country. The government realised that it should form communication links between its largest and most powerful computers, so that if one computer was destroyed, the others could still function. This network was called ARPANET. Very soon, these computers made connections with other computers in other networks and then with international networks and the Internet was born.

Initially, only scientists who had access to mainframe computers used the Internet. However, as technology (and software such as Windows) improved and became more accessible to the general public, the Internet became popular with the general public. Certain protocols became established and a computer language called HTML (hypertext mark-up language) made a graphical (picture based) interface possible. The World-Wide Web (WWW) was born and suddenly the information stored in over 60 million computers was accessible to anybody with a modem and a computer.

The essence of the Internet is communication and the exchange of information. By accessing the world's phone system, it is now possible to exchange documents and files between people or organisations almost anywhere in the world.

Hardware required for connecting to the Internet

Everything about the Internet is slow, because of the limitations of phone lines. It is important to realise that even the fastest Internet connection currently available (ISDN) is slower than the slowest CD-ROM drive. Huge international projects, including using a fibreglass cable network, are aiming to increase this speed so that it approximates current computer speeds.

In the meantime, there are two main factors to consider in order to speed a computer up on the Internet: upgrade the computer so that it works faster or connect to the Internet at quiet times. Upgrading usually means adding more memory, a faster CPU or a faster modem. This will allow the computer to process the information faster. Accessing the Internet at quiet times means more direct routing of telephone calls which speeds up the transfer of information. The best times are when fewer people are using the phone lines: for example, late at night or early in the morning.

The software

Browsers are software programs which can look through the various WWW sites. The user inputs an Internet address and then the program searches through the various connections around the world. When it has found the website it will display the contents on your screen. The two most common browsers are *Internet Explorer* and *Netscape*.

What is a website?

A website is a collection of documents put together by an organisation or an individual. The electronic documents display on the screen as text, pictures, videos, journals, newspapers, music, speech or any other medium of communication. This information is stored on a computer (the server) which is permanently connected to the Internet. Users can access the site by inputting a specific address into their own computer that then connects to the Internet and finds the site.

The address of a website appears quite unusual; for example, 'http://www.natn.org.uk' or 'www.natn.org.uk'. 'http' (hypertext transfer protocol) describes the method used to transfer information from a local computer to a distant computer. This prefix can usually be left out as it is no longer required. 'www' means 'WorldWide Web' and indicates that this is a site on the Web. 'natn' is the name of the organisation, 'org' indicates that an organisation runs the site and 'uk' indicates that it is based in the UK.

Search engines

If the address of a website is unknown, then the Internet can be searched with a program called a 'search engine'. *Alta Vista* is a very popular search engine that is run by a computer manufacturer called Digital.

Searching for article or items on the Internet is a bit like walking through a library; accessing the information is much easier if approached in a logical fashion. Finding articles on perioperative nursing, for example, could involve looking for:

- 'perioperative nursing' – to find articles related to each of these two words. This search is likely to result in around 40 000 articles;
- 'perioperative' and 'nursing' – this will search for individual words and will find around 300 000 articles on 'nursing' and around 4000 articles on 'perioperative';
- 'perioperative nursing' + date + UK – this will limit the search of UK articles from the date when they were written.

Navigating the Web

Once you get to a website, you will probably see the opening screen, called the 'home page'. A typical website might have, for example:

- a home page;
- an information page;
- a subscription page;
- a file library;
- a discussion forum;
- a retail section.

Each one of these pages has a specific address and each can be accessed directly from another page through a series of links. Navigating through a well-constructed website is therefore a series of jumps from one part of the site to another.

A file library might have past documents or articles that you can download on to your own computer for reading at your leisure later. A discussion forum can be used to flag up issues of importance to users of the site or to answer queries and share information. The retail section might sell membership services or products either online or using a fax.

Email

The importance of Internet email is increasing. Faster than the postage system, more versatile than faxing, more permanent than the spoken word, email is fast becoming one of the most important means of communication. email can be used, for example, to send a document, in the form of a word processor file, to any corner of the globe. It can also be used for sending letters, money, pictures, sound, video or any other computer-based item of information.

Sending email is as simple as knowing what a person's email address is; for example, 'editor@natn.org.uk'. This is entered into the email program that you normally find as part of the browser software.

USING THE WORLDWIDE WEB

The Internet is a vast library, crammed full of information and growing at an astounding rate. The WorldWide Web is a collection of Internet sites which make information available in a 'user-friendly' way. The WWW uses all the multimedia features that are available today so an electronic page might contain pictures, videos, sound, text and animation. In plain terms, a page about pressure sores, for example, might contain a video clip illustrating the treatment of pressure sores, a news report and a picture of a scoring tool. These facilities make the WWW an important resource for nurses.

Electronic journals

There are literally hundreds if not thousands of medical and nursing journals on the WWW, many of which offer free access.

Electronic publishing offers several features.

- Interaction with the readers is easy through email.
- Attracting new readers is cheaper and opens up potential new markets at a fraction of the cost of, for example, bulk mailings.
- News stories can be much more timely – as soon as they are published, they can be instantly available to all the readers.
- The Internet has infinite space – 10 years' worth of journals can easily be stored on the Internet.

Journals vary in their content; for example, the *Journal of Obstetrics and Gynaecology Online* (www.ccspublishing.com) is only published on the Internet while the *British Journal of Perioperative Nursing* (www.natn.org.uk) is available in both paper and electronic format.

Access to collections of journals related to nursing and medical issues is available at several sites. For example, Electronic Newsletters and Journals is an alphabetical list which tells you what is available and whether it is available for subscription, free, as a complete journal, etc. This site is at:
www.mfhs.edu/library/webinfo/journal.html
Electronic Publications also do a listing of hundreds of journals at:
www.gen.emory.edu/medweb/alphakey/electronic_publications.html

There are also many hundreds of electronic medical journals available, offering anything from whole journals to abstracts or selected articles. The *Alzheimer's Disease Review*, for example, is a full journal which can be found at:
www.coa.uky.edu/ADReview
The *American Operating Room Nurse's Journal* can be found at:
www.aorn.org
and the *American Journal of Nursing* can be found at:
www.ajn.org/ajn

Medical news

Current medical information can be obtained from various sites: for example, International Medical News at:
www.sma.org/intl/interndx.htm
or Nursing World at:
www.nursingworld.org.connect.htm

Medical sites

There are over 10 000 medical sites on the Internet at present. Most of these sites are free and are supported by advertising. Some are very general and try to offer a 'one-stop site' for all information, but sites which specialise in one area are really superseding this trend.

The Physician's Guide to the Internet is a good starting point because it contains links to other sites. This can be found at:
www.webcom.com.pgi
Those interested in anaesthesiology will find GASNet at:
http://gasnet.med.yale.edu
Cancernet represents oncology at:
www.icic.nci.nih.gov
and surgery can be found at:
www.trauma.org

Medline and CINAHL

Medline and CINAHL will be familiar to most people who have done a literature search in a library. Both these sources of information are indexes of current nursing and medical literature found in journals. They are available in printed and electronic forms but the electronic format is becoming increasingly popular because of the search facilities which this method offers.

CINAHL (Cumulative Index to Nursing and Allied Health Medicine) is produced by the CINAHL Information Systems. It first went online in 1984 and on CD-ROM in 1989. It is now available directly to individuals on the Internet. CINAHL is not free and a charge is made for its use either on CD-ROM or on the Internet. However, libraries and universities often subscribe and offer the service free for their members. CINAHL can be found at:
www.cinahl.com

Medline is a database from the National Library of Medicine (NLM). In April 1996 an Internet version of this program was released in order to facilitate access for research. This service is available for a fee. However, NLM has recently developed a free website called PubMed, which enables the user to search the entire Medline database using Web-based pages. This is available at:
www.ncbi.nlm.nih.gov/PubMed

Medline currently indexes 4000 nursing, medical and health journals with around 8.5 million articles. Perhaps because of these incredible statistics, it is one of the most frequently accessed databases in the world.

There are many other medical databases; for example, a database of autopsy information which lists over 50 000 autopsy reports and 5000 images can be found at:
www.med.jhu.edu/pathology/iad.html

Several thousand clinical trials can be found at:
www.centerwatch.com
and over 3000 terms used for drugs on the streets of Indiana can be found at:
www.drugs.indiana.edu/slang/home.html

Newsgroups

Newsgroups are a useful way of interacting with people who have similar interests. So, for example, a member could send a message to a group of people interested in perioperative nursing asking about pressure area care in the operating room. Someone reads the note, offers some suggestions and sends a reply. Somebody else reads this note and sends an addition with some queries of their own. And so it goes on. This collection of newsgroups is called Usenet and it is organised into groups and subgroups or subjects. There are currently more than 15 000 different Usenet groups covering everything from science and recreation to medicine and physics.

You should be able to access a newsgroup from your browser software but if not, you can use the Internet News program from Microsoft. This is a free program which you can download from CompuServe at:
GO INTEXPLORER
or from Microsoft at:
www.microsoft.com

You will find instruction on how to use the program at these sites. The newsgroups are also free which is a great bonus. A very useful newsgroup can be found at:
News:Sci.med.nursing

HEALTH AND SAFETY ISSUES

As with any tool, there are health hazards associated with the use of a computer. These include eye problems, backache, neckache, headache and repetitive strain injuries.

The screen

A PC monitor uses the same technology, based on a cathode ray tube (CRT), as a normal TV. A CRT is a glass flask, not unlike the inside of a Thermos flask, with three electron guns squirting electrons at a display screen. The radiation is nowhere near as dangerous as gamma rays or X-rays but it can still cause health problems and legislation has recently been introduced in Sweden, in the form of MPR-11 standards, in order to cover this problem. All companies in the UK have to comply with the 1993 Health and Safety (Display Screen Equipment) Regulations that incorporate manufacturing and usage standards.

Eyestrain is another problem because of the proximity of the screen to the user. A flicker-free screen is essential so a monitor with a minimum of 72 Hz refresh rate should be used. The refresh rate (the rate at which the screen redraws itself) can usually be found in the monitor's manual or via the software that came with the graphics card. Screen glare should be kept to a minimum and this can be achieved by turning the screen angle downwards slightly, avoiding working directly underneath bright fluorescent lights or by purchasing an antiglare screen.

Printers

Laser printers produce ozone as the electrostatic charge on the toner drum is released. The ozone is then released into the general environment and in high concentrations is a severe irritant that can cause breathing problems. Modern laser printers produce only about 0.15 mg per 15 minutes and the recommended duration of exposure is 0.6 mg per cubic metre per 15 minutes. Although problems are unlikely to occur, it would be a good precaution to keep an office well ventilated, especially if more than one laser printer is in use.

Toner is another danger from printers. Toner is a very fine dust that is attracted to the charged surface of the laser drum before being melted and 'stuck' to the paper.

Noise pollution is a problem with dot matrix printers. These printers work by striking a ribbon onto the surface of the paper. Some high-speed printers are extremely noisy and irritating and may contribute to stress and other noise-related health problems. If possible, move the printer away from workstations or encase it in a noise-reducing box.

Ergonomics

The posture adopted when using a computer is important. To avoid circulation problems and muscle strain, feet should be kept flat on the floor and a good sitting posture maintained – neither straight upright or slouched down, which puts a strain on the normal contours of the back. Leaning forward and hunching shoulders should be avoided. Taking frequent short rests is better than fewer, longer rests. Ergonomists help employers by devising alternative tasks that let employees move around. It is also possible for a computer to sound an alarm every 30 minutes in order to remind the employee to take a break. While taking a break, stretching the hands, arms and shoulders and neck may help to relax tired muscles.

Carpal tunnel syndrome is a disorder that starts with mild symptoms such as numbness or tingling but can progress to increased pain and loss of dexterity. It might help to keep the wrist in a neutral position and to avoid hitting the keys too hard. Alternatively, consider buying a 'wrist bar' to support the wrists and hands while typing.

Designing an efficient and comfortable workstation should be a priority, especially where a computer is used.

- Plan your workstation for plenty of space.
- Use a comfortable desk chair, on castors with adjustable height.

- Reduce glare from the monitor screen.
- Ensure that the temperature, lighting, humidity and other environmental factors are appropriate.
- Keep noise to a minimum by moving printers, using carpets and other noise-reducing measures.

Further information can be reached via the following websites.
www.sas.ab.ca/biz/christie/safelist.html
http://ergoweb.mech.utah.edu/
www.system-concepts.com/contents_page.html
www.ccta.gov.uk/hse/hsehome.htm

Box 12.2 Glossary

Browser – program for reading documents on the WorldWide Web.

Browsing – wandering through the pages on the Web.

Download – to receive information from somebody else's distant computer to the computer in front of you.

email – electronic mail.

Hardware – the mechanical devices in your computer; for example, a CD-ROM drive.

Internet – a worldwide network of computers which communicate with each other using the same computer language.

Internet service provider – a company which provides access to the Internet.

Modem – a device which converts digital information from a computer into analogue information which can travel over a telephone line.

Search engine – a program which allows you to search for a word or string of words on the WWW.

Software – the programs that make your computer do work.

Upgrade – to install new hardware or software.

Upload – to send information from your own computer to a distant computer.

WorldWide Web – (WWW) the computers and documents on the Internet which are linked together using a visually appealing and user-friendly interface.

Recruitment and retention issues

Adrienne Montgomery

Recruiting and retaining nurses in the operating department has long been debated as a problem. Traditionally, the main source of recruits has been the students who were allocated as 'workers' to the department. During this experience, those students who were thought to have a natural aptitude for perioperative work were nurtured and encouraged to return on registration. On rare occasions an experienced nurse was recruited, often via the recovery room after several years out of nursing practice. Retaining nurses in the operating department was just as simple. For nurses who practised in the operating department, transfer to a ward area was difficult as the department skills were held to be non-transferable and starting again at the bottom was not seen as an attractive alternative for an expert practitioner. Most nurses completed a postregistration nursing course that was often one of the lures to the area. Once captured and safely installed behind closed doors, theatre nurses very rarely escaped, except to another operating department – but this was allowed. The result of this recruitment ploy was a relatively stable workforce with a good skill mix.

In today's competitive world the challenge of recruitment and retention in the operating department threatens the existence of theatre nursing as we know it. The employment and training of technicians of all types to cover staffing shortfalls and in the short term offer an economic staffing solution threatens the traditional role of the theatre nurse, often taking away satisfying aspects of the role. Alongside this is the shift in attitude to the transferability of skills and experienced theatre nurses are taking the opportunity to change career paths. The international trend for fewer people to choose nursing as a career, the numbers of experienced nurses leaving the profession and the greater scope for nursing practice puts theatre nursing in direct competition for scarce professional resources within all areas of nursing. Further complicating the situation are the changes that have occurred in nursing education, where student nurses have little or no exposure to operating department work.

The challenge for managers in the operating department is to approach the issue of recruitment and retention by selling the area as *the* place to practise holistic nursing in an environment which provides support and work excitement. Viewed in this way, recruitment and retention are all about marketing: nurses need to sell perioperative nursing. Factors to consider when marketing a product include the market, the competition, product, strategies and resources. (See Ch 11 for budgeting in the perioperative environment.)

THE MARKET

The market is made up of two groups: experienced registered nurses and newly registered nurses. Both groups have specific needs which must be met if they are to be recruited and retained in perioperative practice. As a consequence, each group requires different marketing strategies.

THE COMPETITION

First, there is the question of whether theatre nursing really is nursing. Theatre nursing is commonly perceived, by those who are not theatre nurses, to be technical, focusing on assisting the surgeon and anaesthetist, rather than focusing on the care of the patient and as such is not 'real' nursing (Johnson 1991, Holmes 1994). In her 1991 study Johnson identified that theatre nurses spent a significant amount of time performing non-nursing tasks, which often take precedence over nursing duties and patient contact. Power (1993) goes so far as to suggest that nurses should give away the scrub nurse role and return to nursing the patient so that the nursing in theatre is visible.

Second, one has to consider the career choices open to nurses today. The roles available to nurses have evolved with the changes in the health-care system and nurse education. Upward of 60 career choices within nursing can be identified, of which theatre nursing is but one. For the newly registered nurse the career choices available are more extensive than in the past. It has been identified that graduates of college-based nursing programmes experiment with areas of practice (Montgomery 1985). They choose to work for limited periods of 3–12 months in different specialities, usually beginning with the more general before selecting the specialist areas that demand a more in-depth knowledge for practice. This generalist to specialist pattern is usually guided by the need to enter specialist areas with some predetermined level of experience.

The choice of area is also influenced by the experiences gained as students. Research tells us that certain clinical situations are perceived as difficult, challenging and/or stressful for nursing students (Cooke 1996). Practice experience becomes difficult or a challenge when technical skills are involved and when the expectations of the registered nurses in the area are not congruent with the students' level of knowledge and practice. Also, if the attitude of staff in the practice area is perceived to be antagonistic to students, the degree of difficulty and stress increases.

Crofts & Taylor (1996) identified seven factors that make the students' operating department experience stressful. For example, fear of the unknown – what really happens behind the closed doors? Fear of the reaction to the surgical procedure is a stressful experience: the 'Will I faint?'

thing, usually founded on horror stories traditionally passed on from one group of students to another. Lack of patient contact is seen as stressful; presumably this arises from a perceived view of what theatre nursing is. It is stressful for students when there is a lack of recognition of their vulnerability. For the student who does receive more experience than a patient follow-through, task orientation, being a part of a skilled workforce and the associated need to develop instant skills, and the lack of support are all seen to be stressful. The greater the stress level for the students, the more likely it is that the theatre experience will be perceived as unpleasant. Thus the likelihood of these students choosing the operating department as an area for practice on registration is negligible.

For registered nurses, not only the changes in the health-care system but role redefinition, higher patient/nurse ratios and lack of recognition are all factors that influence their decision to either change their career paths or leave nursing altogether. For this group, theatre nursing is rarely considered as an option. It is either viewed as part of the high-stress, acute care area they seek to leave or it is not real nursing. For the experienced theatre nurse, the decision to leave the area is influenced by the sharing of the nurse's role with operating department practitioners and the perceived reduction in role satisfaction.

THE PRODUCT

The product for sale is the exciting work of the perioperative nurse. The work nurses do in the operating department is clearly defined and significant when measured against patient outcomes.

Theatre nursing provides:

- a fast pace;
- visible patient improvement;
- respect for knowledge;
- people contact;
- research;
- challenging projects;
- knowledge that one is making a difference to patient outcomes;
- variety;
- team membership;
- teaching and learning;
- assessment;
- the growth of others;
- high-acuity patients.

Nurses entering or remaining in the area need a variety of experiences, opportunity to try management skills, suitable working conditions and arrangements, challenges, the chance to be creative, accountability and clinical leadership, all of which are the ingredients needed for work excitement. Work excitement is personal enthusiasm and commitment that is demonstrated in creativity, teaching and learning and taking opportunities in everyday situations (Lickmann et al 1993). It is work excitement that will sell theatre nursing and successfully recruit and retain nurses. Taking each aspect of theatre nurses' work, we have the selling points for a recruitment campaign. At the same time, involvement of experienced theatre nurses in the recruitment process provides new challenges and promotes work excitement and thus reduces the risk of these nurses seeking to move to other areas of nursing.

RECRUITMENT STRATEGIES

Variety is found in the range of roles the nurse may take, such as advocate, infection control monitor, safety officer, team leader, scrub nurse, postoperative intensive care, teacher, learner and more. Each role represents a dimension of nursing care provided in the area. No day in the operating theatre is ever the same as the next. Even when working in a particular speciality within the department, the variety of operations and different make-up of the team from list to list provide variety so that routine is never boring or predictable.

While on an organisational level working conditions are dictated by employment contracts and policy, at the departmental level they are ordered by rosters, personnel and quality breaks. More importantly, the working conditions are ordered by the philosophies and values articulated by the department which define and model the practice and quality of patient care.

The arrangement of work in the operating department is unique and the independent role of the nurse is the catalyst for work excitement. The interdisciplinary nature of the team, each member interdependent on the other to carry out their independent role function, and the focus on the patient as central are not found in such a pure form in other areas of nursing. The independent role function affords the nurse control and accountability for quality patient care.

Challenge and creativity arise out of the learning environment theatre work provides. The high-tech atmosphere and fast pace of work offer the nurse learning opportunities with each patient that both motivate and stimulate. The nature of each patient encounter challenges existing knowledge that allows the nurse to design individual care – no two 'total hip replacements' will ever be the same!

The work excitement that exists in theatre nursing is the marketing tool to be used in meeting the challenge of recruitment and retention in the operating theatre. The way this tool is used determines the success or failure of a manager's endeavours and is dependent on the commitment of all theatre nurses to make it work.

It is imperative that any strategy for recruitment is planned to include financial and human resources (see Box 13.1). All staff must be involved in planning and implementing the recruitment campaign. Ownership of the campaign ensures success and becomes in itself a retention strategy.

Box 13.1	Strategies for recruitment
Planning	
Resources	
Ownership by all staff	

New graduates	*Experienced RNs*
Advertising	Advertising
Virtual tours	Real-life tours
Introductory course	Introductory course
Relationship with nursing school	In-service education
Team approach to perioperative care	

Involvement brings to the fore respect for knowledge, people contact, research, teamwork, challenge, teaching and learning, growth of self and others and the long-term outcome of making a difference to patient outcomes. All these ingredients ensure work excitement. Each staff member brings a talent that is identified and developed.

To ensure that staff are comfortable participating in a recruitment campaign, depending on the extent and type of campaign, workshops may be held to prepare and develop the strategies, resources and roles they may take. Time must be planned into the working hours for the development of resources as required. When looking to recruit staff who are experienced in other areas of nursing, it is important to establish what type of operating department experience they did or did not have as students and identify their perception of what perioperative nursing is. The findings of this research provide the approach to be taken to the recruitment.

When recruiting qualified staff, one can dip into two pools of personnel. The first is found outside the organisation and the second within the organisation. Three strategies are outlined here and may be used for either group, but it is important to identify clearly which is to be the target of a campaign.

Advertising

Advertising is the most common form of recruitment; when it is employed the work excitement must be highlighted. This will include the working conditions and arrangements, variety and learning opportunities. Always invite personal contact from the enquirer – the personal touch in selling your department can never be overestimated. If your agency has a website, arrange for a virtual tour through the department to be set up. The tour will introduce the potential recruits to the layout of the department and personnel and the unique and important features are highlighted.

Team building

Team building is the second strategy that can be employed. The team is made up of personnel employed in the operating department and those in the pre- and postoperative areas that have a common goal of individualised evidence-based care for the patients. Preoperative visiting is an ideal but not always possible for day surgery and emergency patients. The alternative is the development of model plans for care, based on evidence, by representatives of each area and individualised for each patient. These plans go beyond which bit is to be shaved and the fasting regime to involve assessment of anxiety, anticipated pain response and patients' knowledge of procedure, expectations of the surgical experience and more. Working together in this way enhances the team members' knowledge and understanding of each other and engenders collegiality. It also opens the door for potential recruits to come into the operating department and operating personnel to share in pre- and postoperative care. How this experience is set up determines whether or not ward personnel will be tempted to join the team.

Operating department personnel can take the initiative to inform the ward nurses by hosting education sessions, either in the department or outside. Examples of sessions might be predicting pain response, the physiological effects of surgery, specific operative procedures, infection control or patient safety. Resources to assist these sessions should be developed, including handouts for future reference. The increased understanding of the operative phase improves patient outcomes and acts as a lure to come into the department and learn more.

Encouraging staff to follow patients through the operative phase is central to this strategy. It is important that staff coming into the department are given realistic expectations of the time commitment and involvement in patient care. Providing visitors with comprehensive written information guides their knowledge development and directs them to focus on patient care, not just the operation. Taking time to develop the information sheets and setting them out in a standard format that identifies all aspects of care as headings, e.g. infection control, safety, pain management, effects of positioning, will assist in explicating the roles, especially if each team member's role is identified. The compendium of information sheets then forms the basis of a handbook for new recruits and is an example of audit evidence for staff development. During the theatre visit, a 'buddy' should be assigned to support, guide and involve the visitor in the patient care.

No operating department experience is complete without a debriefing session. This allows for questions arising out of reflection on the experience to be addressed and an invitation for another visit to be issued. The success of the visit will determine whether or not the person is tempted back for more.

Introduction courses

The third strategy is to offer an introduction to the operating department course, the purpose of which is to provide an overview of theatre work and enough knowledge of procedure and process to function safely at a novice level in the operating department. The course may be set up jointly with the local college or be an in-house course. An example of such a course would be 18 hours in length, run for 3 hours over 6 weeks in the evening or over 2 days at the weekend. The course would take place in the operating department and involve an introduction to procedures and processes. The opportunity to scrub and don gown and gloves and assist with simulated cases and familiarisation with and handling of equipment are included. Advertising vacancies at the same time as advertising the course is a positive initiative in the recruitment of individuals who have thought of trying the operating department but are not sure of making the move. The staff involved in teaching the course must have this activity planned into their workload.

Capturing the interest of students requires developing a relationship with the local school of nursing. The relationship with the school can involve research and education as well as student experience. The closer the relationship, the more positive the results. Working together to provide the best experience for the students, even if it is just one visit to follow a patient through, may be enough to tempt them back when qualified. The structured process for the students on a follow-through visit is the same as that employed for qualified personnel who visit the department. For students fortunate enough to be allocated to the operating department, a structured experience is required, tailored to the length of experience and availability of a clinical teacher. If the school of nursing has some ownership of the course, students may well be able to complete the course as part of their preregistration nursing programme.

RETENTION STRATEGIES

Work excitement can also be used as a basis for retention strategies. Each of these predictors has to be addressed in relation to each staff member as they all have their own interpretation of what makes work exciting.

Variety does not necessarily mean moving from one area to another – for example, theatre to recovery – although this may provide some staff with enough variety. It means broadening the role so that it is more than the obvious. Some may take on some management duties alongside the duties of an operative team member. For others, it may be quality control or teaching students. The identification of each staff member's preference is part of the appraisal process and professional development.

Providing good working conditions includes considering the needs of the person as rosters are drawn up which assures staff members that they are valued and that other aspects of life that impact on work are as important as turning up for a shift. Quality breaks are needed to ensure a refreshed staff, no matter how short that break may be. The facilities available for the comfort of staff and the environment in general should foster collegiality. How personnel interact is fundamental to the smooth running of the department and to ensuring they stay. The working conditions are ultimately ordered by the philosophies and values articulated by the

Box 13.2 Retention strategies	
Planning	
Resources	
Ownership by all staff	
Variety of roles	Working conditions
Change and challenge	Philosophies and values
Team building	Professional development

department which define and model practice within the operating department. If the working conditions are to allow each member to grow and develop in the provision of quality patient care, all staff must own the philosophies and values.

Change as a predictor of work excitement is inherent within the work of the theatre personnel. No two days are the same, team membership changes within a day and thus the routine is never boring – or so it might seem. While having variety in one's work reduces the sameness, having the same activities over time means that the work will become predictable. Changing the activities puts the novelty and challenge back into the work, for it is the challenge that change creates that stimulates the excitement. Change is planned and owned by the staff as it arises out of the identified needs of each individual and is implemented in a challenging but non-threatening way.

Growth and development occur in a setting where learning opportunities are provided, valued and maximised. Four variables are identified as representing learning opportunities in the work environment (Lickmann et al 1993). They are the availability of opportunity, a high-tech atmosphere, a motivating and stimulating environment and working with other health professionals. The operating department provides all these factors so the failure of any one individual to grow professionally is unlikely, but it can happen. The value placed on professional development is the foundation for growth of individuals and the department. Actively supporting research initiatives and conference attendance as either presenter or participant are ways that overtly support development, whereas change and variety covertly support learning.

CONCLUSION

For recruitment and retention strategies to be successful, they have to be planned and implemented deliberately. Resources, human and financial, have to be allocated. But, most importantly, the staff in the department must own the strategies. The strategies must address the competition and sell perioperative nursing as patient-centred and exciting work in which both new recruits and existing staff grow and are fulfilled.

REFERENCES

Cooke M 1996 Nursing students' perceptions of difficult or challenging clinical situations. Journal of Advanced Nursing 24(6): 1281–1287

Crofts L, Taylor M 1996 A new model for Project 2000 students in theatre. British Journal of Nursing 5(3): 136–144

Holmes L 1994 Theatre nursing (part 1). British Journal of Theatre Nursing 5(5): 11–15

Johnson G 1991 Scrubbing – a sacred cow. Nursing 4(43): 19–21

Lickman P, Simms L, Green C 1993 Learning environment: the catalyst for work excitement. Journal of Continuing Education in Nursing 25(5): 211–217

Montgomery A 1985 Retention survey. Auckland Hospital Board, New Zealand

Power K 1993 Role over? Nursing Times 89(41): 72, 75

Excellence in perioperative practice

Marilyn Williams

I do not pretend to teach her how, I ask her to teach herself, and for this purpose I venture to give her some hints. (Florence Nightingale, 1859)

Miss Nightingale seems to be telling us that nursing is a practice-based discipline, in which those who seek to become skilled must take responsibility for their own learning, listen to and emulate their peers. The pathway to excellence in practice begins with and relies upon this sense of personal responsibility.

DEFINING EXCELLENCE

Defining excellence is not easy. It is a concept which, like art, is probably more easily recognised than defined in understandable terms. Conway (1996) refers to expert practice, expertise, specialist and advanced practice. All of these contribute to excellence and no single term provides a sufficient definition. Excellence in nursing practice is a subjective and contextually related concept, probably best appreciated when observing experienced nurses working seemingly on autopilot – doing exactly the right thing at the right time, anticipating, responding, reacting and all without conscious thought or effort. Benner (1984) identifies this beautifully as 'the passage from detached observer to involved performer'.

DEVELOPING EXCELLENCE

Becoming an accomplished perioperative practitioner is a learning process which for most nurses is not a conscious experience. People learn in their own way and at their own rate. The theories which support this are based in psychology, a behavioural science now well established in nurse education. As well as the behavioural approach, in which learning takes place, is remembered and recalled for use, the humanistic learning theories have other dimensions:

The first is that of teaching subject matter in a more human way, that is facilitating subject matter learning by students. The second is that of educating the non-intellectual or affective aspects of the student . . . developing persons who understand themselves, who understand . . . and can relate to others. (Patterson 1973)

Developing excellence in perioperative practitioners demands the humanistic approach. Where nursing care takes place in a highly structured and technologically complex environment, it would be easy to lose both nurse and patient in the machinery. Meeting the human needs of patients during their perioperative care is a powerful basis for practice. Understanding yourself and relating to patients and to others around you is a sound basis for developing excellence and becoming a reflective practitioner can be a useful part of this process (Conway 1998).

EXPERIENTIAL LEARNING

The second most potent learning influence is experience. Experience is the concrete reality of doing something and learning through that doing. Student nurses and teachers in a study by Burnard (1992) declared that experiential learning was 'learning by doing, personal learning, [and] it involves reflection'. Reflection combines the art and science of nursing, where experiences in practice are made personal for the learner and, as Conway's (1998) study found, 'the process of reflection was seen as central to learning from practice and developing knowledge in the practice setting'.

Nurses, although possibly unable to state the rules and rationales for their clinical practices, are nevertheless in possession of tacit and intuitive knowledge (James & Clarke 1994) acquired from experiences. This inability to express such knowledge may mean that it is not recognised or valued and for this reason we must respond to Glen's (1995) implication 'for nursing education to be based more firmly in the reality of practice'.

Experience coupled with formal structured education does not necessarily result in successful learning. A study by Daley (1997) indicates other important influences:

> Findings indicate that nurses used information from continuing education programmes to construct a knowledge base and that this process was affected by the structural, human resources, political and symbolic frames of the context in which nurses practise.

The relationship of context to knowledge and practice was also found in Conway's (1998) study, which not only examined what nurses said they did but also observed what they actually did and revealed inconsistencies between the two.

INFLUENCES ON LEARNING

On this author's questioning of theatre nurses about their careers and the ways in which they learned, some interesting observations were made. Role models appear to be important, as do structure, organisation and discipline. When asked about the significance of discipline, a theatre nurse said: 'I think it's an essential factor in nursing, and especially in theatres, because without structure and discipline, it doesn't matter what area you work in . . . because without that basic foundation you've got nothing to build on'. This response reflects the controlled and controlling nature of theatres as a clinical setting. There are rules and usually only one right way of doing things. As nurses learn the rules and right ways, a feeling of security in practice and a competent technical performance is the likely result. Whilst accepting that this is a valuable learning pathway, being allowed to make mistakes and learn from them has to be part of it. This requires patience and tolerance on the part of the person who is guiding the learner.

This emphasis on performance is not without its critics. Milligan (1998) points out that a focus on technical skills debases the concept of educating and empowering students to become critical thinkers delivering holistic care. Le Var (1996) examined National Vocational Qualifications, which are largely performance based, in the context of nursing and midwifery education and found the assessment process to be 'bureaucratic, reductionist and fragmented in nature and unlikely to engender analysis and synthesis'. This puts vocational programmes and qualifications conceptually at odds with the university-based preparation of nurses but this is redeemable through the processes of APL (accreditation of prior learning), APA (accreditation of prior achievement) and APEL (accreditation of prior experiential learning) which universities offer as a means of access to courses and awards (Williams 1996).

This system is probably the answer for the theatre nurse who, when asked about current nurse education, said:

The way it is today, it's not compatible with how I see nursing . . . the health service has changed such a lot in 50 years, some areas it's expanded and it's moved on, in other areas it's lost its direction . . . I think nurses have been misled over the last 15–20 years, in that they have been led . . . in the wrong direction.

This nurse felt that theory had become more important than practice and that practice was no longer valued. In fact, the university system does provide nurses with opportunities to develop practice expertise and practising nurses are currently the guardians of the standards to which that practice is taught and assessed. This is a significant responsibility for which currently practising nurses are accountable, though many who are quick to criticise students and the education process do not admit or acknowledge their part in it.

Developing expertise in practice is influenced by the clinical learning environment. What makes a clinical environment an effective place to learn was the subject of a study by Hart & Rotem (1995). They found six influencing factors which positively influenced professional development: 'role clarity, autonomy and recognition, job satisfaction, quality of supervision, peer support and opportunities for learning'.

The same theatre nurse quoted above, when asked what was the right direction for nurse education, said: 'The right direction is the direction that you personally want to go, it's very individual, it's maybe very selfish . . .

education has led nurses in a direction which I don't think was very beneficial'. This seems to fit with Hart & Rotem's (1995) findings, with an emphasis on the development of the individual, rather than formal teaching and qualifications, and Kolb's (1984) description of learning as 'the process whereby knowledge is created by the transformation of experience'. The nurse's experience, the researchers' findings and the accepted theory all point to the personal nature of the process. While personal development is a satisfying and rewarding process for the individual, the universities have to produce competent and professional nurses in sufficient numbers to sustain the NHS and to a standard which will meet the requirement for registration laid down by the UKCC. In this case, the needs of the NHS and the UKCC inevitably take precedence over those of the individual.

ROLE MODELS AND THE TEAM

A theatre sister with 10 years' experience rated team working and 'team spirit' as important attributes to both job satisfaction and learning: 'We rely very heavily on each other to do each other's jobs confidently, and also with a sense of humour'. When asked for significant incidents related to learning in theatre, this sister said:

> Admiring senior people, thinking 'one day I want to be like that', and picking out what I thought were the qualities in each of these people, really learning from their experiences and their mistakes, and my own, obviously because only time and experience really make you experienced, more confident and more competent, it's just an ever increasing circle.

The critical role played by a respected senior role model for this sister and the self-development described are in keeping with 'recent developments in nursing, which focus on learning from experience and utilise the concept of the reflective practitioner to inform their various models' (Mallik 1998).

A very experienced G grade sister, when asked how she learned in theatre, instantly responded, 'Role models, the theatre superintendent, the senior theatre sisters, who were much older than me, and also my peers'. When asked if surgeons had played any part in her learning, she replied, 'Yes, I learned how to behave in theatre, not from their behaviour, but what they expected from me, what I knew they expected from me, and from the older more experienced surgeons, and anaesthetists, I learned what they would accept from me'. This account is entirely in keeping with this nurse's age and background. She was trained when behavioural objectives (Quinn 1988) – visible changes in students' behaviour as a result of learning – produced nurses who were obedient, subservient, rule adhering and compliant. Quinn (1988) goes on to point out that the major changes in nurse education recently have all been accepted 'without a trace of industrial action or protest' and he 'makes this point because nurses have always had a tendency to undervalue their abilities and achievements and this has a bearing on the process of change and innovation in the nursing curriculum'. This subservient and submissive response is eloquently described by the nurse above.

Knowing what is expected of you and of others in theatre shows how operating department staff are interdependent. The nurse looked to her peers and the surgeons for guidance on acceptable behaviours to emulate and also as a source of learning. An experienced senior lecturer recalled her days as a theatre nurse by acknowledging the role of operating department assistants in teaching and providing role models for nurses. She said:

> *I was amazed by what they knew, before I went to work in theatre I had no idea they existed, and at first I thought they just did the anaesthetics and the cleaning! I soon found out differently and was very grateful for their help in teaching me and showing me the ropes.*

This example shows clearly the importance of teamwork.

A PERSONAL PATHWAY TO THEATRE

A theatre sister of nearly 30 years' experience related her story of becoming a theatre nurse 'by accident'. She was working part time on a children's ward in a small specialised neurosurgical hospital. The ward was to be closed and the children transferred to the local children's hospital. A new theatre was being built at the neurosurgical hospital at that time and this nurse was offered the opportunity to work in theatre, 'to see if she liked it'. When asked how long it took to decide whether she liked it, she replied, 'From the first week, I got a buzz from it because I was made to feel worthy. . . I felt satisfaction from the work I did on the ward, but not as great as I felt in theatre; my self-esteem shot up'. This was the start of a lifelong personal devotion to neurosurgery, which has given this nurse a very personally rewarding career. She had previously spent 3 months in theatres, on nights, during her training. She admits to loving this experience too, even though she admits, 'I suppose we were thrown in at the deep end, but then the culture was you got on with it, you used your common sense, and you learned to be practical very quickly if you weren't already'.

This emphasis on skilled performance is certainly one which the author can relate to and its importance cannot be underestimated. Patients expect nurses to be able to do their job and do it well. In an operating department context, the other members of the team expect everyone to be able to do their job well, as a failing member will let the team down. Quinn (1988) recognises this in stating that nurses must 'possess a wide variety of skills that demand physical ability and coordination' and this is very apparent in operating departments.

THEORY AND PRACTICE COMBINED

The teaching and learning of nursing skills cannot be separated from the cognitive knowledge which supports it, otherwise it becomes 'rote learning' (Quinn 1988), a simple reproduction of memorised patterns which the learner cannot explain the meaning or significance of. This is not compatible with the autonomous professional practitioner which being a qualified nurse represents. Studdy et al (1994) offer an integrated skills teaching model which they produced to meet:

> ... the needs of students in the light of changes in health care provision and nurse education. By providing opportunities within the curriculum for the development of sound clinical skills, the student nurse is able to develop into the knowledgeable doer described by the UKCC.

It is interesting to note that the same model is used for teaching clinical skills to doctors (Studdy et al 1994) and that multiprofessional shared learning is becoming increasingly common.

IT HELPS IF YOU ENJOY IT!

Job satisfaction is an important influence on developing expertise in practice. A theatre sister who is also an RMN decided that although she enjoyed psychiatric nursing, her change of career was prompted by the feeling that she 'couldn't offer these patients what they really needed' and having enjoyed her theatre allocation as a student nurse, elected to make her career there. The sister with nearly 30 years' experience declares:

> I've had a good living from it, it's not just the monetary issues, it's what it did for me as a person, I've had some very good highs, but I've also had some bad lows, but it taught me to cope with it . . . I've been very lucky, but I put it down to the people who, in the old days I suppose, that I was brought up with . . . I've also put a lot of myself into it, I feel I've given one hundred per cent.

This nurse also offered the opinion that if she gave the surgeon sound and efficient service, then the surgeon likewise would be able to give the patient a better service than if the nurse was struggling or failing. Perhaps some of this nurse's satisfaction with her work came from delivering good patient care by proxy.

There is an implicit realisation in these nurses' accounts that learning is a continuous process, which goes on largely unconsciously most of the time. Learning from basic preregistration education or formal postbasic courses does not figure in these accounts as the nurses describe their learning from a purely practice point of view. This begs the question of which learning experiences are significant and useful for practising nurses. Daley (1997) made this the subject of a research study, which found that 'the role of continuing education and staff development is facilitating a process of learning, reflection, growth and change'. This is a far cry from the behavioural and subservient approach described by Quinn (1988). It is significant that the person is now valued as a learner, encouraged to disclose what they already know and discover what they need to know. Daley (1997) also observes that nurse managers and teachers should be involved in deciding with learners what opportunities are most valuable to them and this is supported by Williams (1996).

There is another side to using experience as a learning tool as Downs (1995) points out:

> *Experience, being the culmination of past learning, is a great help in learning something new, but can also be a major hindrance . . . the hindrance comes when we are unwilling to see beyond our experience and either reject the new or distort it to fit our experience.*

Most perioperative nurses will have met people who are so set in their ways that they reject or ignore anything new, often to the detriment of their practice. These entrenched attitudes may also be reflected in responses to any attempt to change practice, even in response to validated research. Nurses who have attended courses and perhaps obtained academic awards or specialist qualifications are often faced with an uphill struggle or outright resentment when trying to put their new knowledge into practice. Newly qualified nurses with diploma or degree qualifications may also encounter resentment and criticism from experienced staff who do not understand, and do not want to understand, new approaches to nursing.

BAD TIMES CAN BE GOOD FOR YOU!

Even the stress of working in the operating department was seen by a theatre sister as a positive learning experience. The ability to adapt rapidly to changing circumstances, to be able to think on your feet, reorganise yourself and others are stressful but inescapable necessities of life in the operating department and can be valuable. She recounts that:

> *Coming in [on call] in the middle of the night, to a patient with an extradural [haematoma], who's desperately, desperately ill, and within a couple of hours you've done a really good job, with the senior registrar who's probably been up the night before as well, but you've organised it, you've done it and that patient's going to be well.*

This is in keeping with Kolb's (1984) statement that 'Immediate personal experience is the focal point for learning, giving life, texture and subjective personal meaning to abstract concepts and at the same time providing a concrete publicly shared reference point' and this nurse's account bears this out.

Another nurse tells how she conquered her fear of one particular procedure by mentally taking the operation apart and going through the instrument set used for it. By examining the related anatomy and the instruments and by close observation of the surgeon, the nurse became accomplished at assisting with this procedure which, although it had been done for many years in her unit, had remained unpopular with many of the nurses. It was regarded as a difficult and technically awkward procedure. She said, 'I felt frustrated that I could not figure this procedure out so that I understood it to my own satisfaction'. The surgeon who did this operation was very good at it; it is a risky procedure and the surgeon's frustration with less than efficient assistance was often expressed. The situation was not helped by having old and not fully compatible instruments. The turning point for this nurse came with the purchase of a new and fully integrated set of instruments. The surgeon's delight at his new 'toys' was obvious and the nurse privately resolved to 'get to grips' with the procedure. This was duly accomplished and proved very satisfying for both surgeon and nurse. Being able to offer skilled and efficient assistance to surgeons is an important contribution to team building, inspiring confidence and satisfaction.

TEAMWORK

'The whole is greater than the sum of the parts. Teams can achieve by working together what individuals cannot possibly achieve on their own' (Harris 1996). Perioperative practice represents a clear example of teamwork but the people who make up the team bring with them 'massively different prior experiences, even when apparently they might have a similar background, [this] influences the knowledge which they can be assumed to have' (Boud & Walker 1992).

Simply putting a group of people together and expecting them to work effectively as a team is a rash assumption, as Rushin et al (1998) point out. Effective teams can truly transform a department, leading to vastly improved job satisfaction, lower staff sickness and turnover and a better service to patients (Davidson 1998). Ideally, 'Teams are cooperative groups where members acknowledge others members' contributions . . . In principle, teamwork is non-hierarchical and power is shared' (Bond 1998). In practice, this ideal is not always realised and people have to work together as best they can regardless of conflicts, hierarchies and abuse of power. Such difficulties often manifest themselves in the form of a 'sacred cows' – 'an object or tradition which is held in such popular esteem that it is considered to be above criticism – even justified criticism' (Shukmaker 1996 cited by Wicker 1997). Well-established teams may be resentful towards new members who suggest alternatives or attempt to change these sacred cows.

Becoming a member of a team nearly always involves individuals making personal adjustments to fit in with others. Rarely do teams make changes to fit in with individuals, unless that individual has the authority and specific remit to change the team. Teamwork is increasingly seen as essential for successful patient care in all environments but to be successful the team must be supported by an appropriate management style and organisational culture (Baxter 1997, Bond 1998). Such things cannot be taken for granted in operating departments.

ROLE IDENTITIES

Just as nursing itself is not clearly defined, perioperative nursing also suffers from the lack of a clear identity. The question of what perioperative nurses do is often asked and much debate ensues about the answers. Baxter (1996) offers the most sensible answer; following the National Association of Theatre Nurses' (NATN) review of the role of the perioperative nurse she and they concluded that the role of the perioperative nurse was the same as that of any nurse in any part of an acute hospital. This means assessing, planning, delivering and evaluating care for patients. Baxter (1996) adds significantly, 'The fact that the nurse provides skilled assistance to the surgeon and anaesthetist does not diminish that role'. So the answer is quite clear: nurses in operating departments nurse patients through the processes of anaesthesia, surgery and recovery, providing appropriate and safe care and documenting that care and being accountable for it. For nurses this is the end of the matter; for surgeons and anaesthetists, the answer may be different.

The author asked consultant anaesthetists and surgeons what they expected from theatre nurses and 'caring for patients' was not prominent in their answers. They want nurses to organise and manage the operating departments, lists and workload for them. One surgeon said he would not greatly miss nurses in theatre, as long as the work was managed efficiently 'so as not to waste time'!! The response from consultant anaesthetists was similar. The widely held view was that as long as they had skilled assistance for anaesthetic induction, maintenance and monitoring, it didn't really matter who provided it. Recovery was the only area seen by surgeons and anaesthetists as one where nursing was required. Observation of recovery areas confirms the impression that once surgery is completed, surgeons and anaesthetists are content to hand over patients to nurses' care and proceed with the next case. This situation is perhaps the impetus behind the movement to expand the role of theatre nurses into a 'perioperative' domain, where nurses meet patients before surgery, lead preassessment clinics and follow up patients after surgery (Cogman 1997). Such arrangements would certainly be much more in keeping with the holistic and humanistic concepts which underpin current nurse education in both pre- and postregistration courses.

Even more adventurous expansion of the nurse's role into anaesthesia (MacRae 1996, Preston 1996) and surgery (Erickson 1996) has already taken place and been enthusiastically received by those involved. Wicker (1996) expresses his concerns that such diversions may in fact represent a fragmentation rather than an enhancement of the nurse's role and, bearing in mind Baxter's (1996) already quoted assertion, these are valid concerns. Perioperative nursing already has natural divisions which may be the cause of conflict.

SPECIALISATION

From common foundations nursing has evolved into many specialisms. Perioperative nursing lends itself to natural divisions – anaesthesia, surgery and recovery – and some nurses have elected to develop their expertise within one specialist role. There is nothing wrong with this. Such an arrangement has worked extremely well for medicine. It can be argued that patients get a better service from highly specialist nurses who practise in a single role but the counter argument of fragmented care can also be applied, as discussed above. On the other hand, managers may want a flexible workforce of 'all-rounders' and so expect perioperative nurses to be able to function in any part of the care environment. In some units anaesthesia care has become the exclusive province of ODAs and ODPs, with nurses delivering intraoperative and recovery care. Overcoming such well-established demarcation lines to produce a workforce who are all-rounders would be a major task.

Successful development of excellence in perioperative practice must make a happy marriage – or at least an amicable friendship – between the technical demands of anaesthesia and surgery and the caring and nurturing expected of nurses. Both are examined, compared and analysed by Varona (1997) who demonstrates, with incidents from practice, the influence of caring and nurturing in combination with technical knowledge. Erickson (1996) was instrumental in initiating a nurse-as-surgeon service for minor procedures at her hospital. Far from fragmenting care, she declares her new role gives her increased contact with patients: 'I see them before operating, counselling them about their operation and giving them advice on postoperative care'. Very few surgical patients would have such supportive nursing care before, during and after surgery organised on more traditional lines. These are two examples of extremely successful specialisation within perioperative nursing. There are many more in the literature (Ferguson 1995, Hood 1995, MacRae 1996, Preston 1996). Perhaps the crux of the debate about perioperative nursing roles and specialisation lies not in analysing what individual nurses do but in ensuring the holistic nature of care, where every nurse, regardless of role, respects and responds to the uniqueness of each patient and cares for them accordingly.

THE ROLE OF MANAGEMENT IN DEVELOPING EXPERTISE

'The microcosm of management represented by a clinical area, ward, department or operating department may be a significant example of the influence of one person' (Williams 1995). Whilst appreciating teamwork and contributions of individuals, much of what happens in an operating department is the result of management and, with it, organisational culture. The management dimensions which bring about change, development, progress or the maintenance of the status quo are power and influence. Handy (1993) explains that:

> *Power and influence make up the fine texture of organisations, and indeed all interactions. Influence is the process whereby A seeks to modify the attitudes or behaviour of B. Power is that which enables him to do it.*

Conway (1996) makes an eloquent case for management support of nurses with some moving critical incidents from her research study, whilst Webster (1996) shares her experiences of managing difficult situations. All are testimony to the role of management in all aspects of staff performance and development. Most nurses in operating departments are only too well aware of the management's role and policy as it affects them. The rules – written or unwritten – on what happens in a particular department are probably as much the result of cultural evolution as direct policy. This situation may be good, bad or somewhere in between.

In order to best serve the workforce, management must know them and be aware of their needs. Expressions of gratitude, sympathy or support at the requisite time go a long way towards making people feel wanted and valued (Williams 1997). Handy (1993) defined managers' roles as leading, administering and fixing and most of a manager's workload will fall within these broad divisions. He goes on to say that managers may also act as a 'GP' to the workforce, diagnosing problems and prescribing treatments. This could certainly be seen as administering and fixing. However managers see their roles, in order to get the best from the workforce, honesty, openness and willingness to listen are essential. There will inevitably be times when workforce requests cannot be granted or when the manager has to be the bearer of bad news. The outcomes of such situations will be greatly influenced by the management style and organisational culture. Creating an environment where expertise and excellence can develop would be a glowing testimony to any manager.

EXCELLENCE IN PRACTICE

Those who wish to become recognised as expert and excellent practitioners must set out to become so by their own efforts. Conway (1996) found that expert nurses whom she categorised as humanistic existentialists were '. . . passionate about nursing. They were politically aware and capable of devising strategies to enable them to develop their practice. They were also very aware of the influence they had on other nurses'. All these characteristics were referred to by the nurses whose experiences were shared earlier in this chapter.

It is undoubtedly easier to develop excellence in practice where the management and organisational culture are supportive, but individual nurses can overcome many obstacles if they are determined to do so. This may involve changing jobs to find the environment that will foster them, seeking out and paying for education to support practice and making some personal commitment to study, improve and learn. The nurses who shared their experiences with the author all seemed to have the 'passion for nursing' which Conway referred to. They had all worked in theatre for many years and still loved it in spite of many things which they wished were different. There is something very special about this type of nursing which is impossible to put into words but which perioperative nurses instinctively know and respond to positively. Maybe these are the potential seeds of excellence.

REFERENCES

Baxter B 1996 The role of the nurse in theatres. British Journal of Theatre Nursing 5(11): 5–7

Baxter B 1997 Operating department staffing – a business manager's perspective. British Journal of Theatre Nursing 7(7): 11–17

Benner P 1984 From novice to expert. Excellence and power in clinical nursing practice. Addison-Wesley, California

Bond P 1998 Teamwork in healthcare – time for review. British Journal of Theatre Nursing 8(4): 19–24

Boud D, Walker D 1992 In the midst of experience: developing a model to aid learners and facilitators. In: Mulligan J, Griffin C (eds) Empowerment through experiential learning. Explorations of good practice. Kogan Page, London

Burnard P 1992 Learning from experience: nurse tutors' and student nurses' perceptions of experiential learning: some initial findings. International Journal of Nursing Studies 29(2): 151–161

Cogman C 1997 A diploma in perioperative practice for the millennium? Open forum. British Journal of Theatre Nursing 6(11): 10

Conway J E 1996 Nursing expertise and advanced practice. Quay Books, Salisbury

Conway J E 1998 Evolution of the species 'expert nurse'. An examination of the practical knowledge held by expert nurses. Journal of Clinical Nursing 7: 75–82

Daley B J 1997 Creating mosaics: the interrelationships of knowledge and context. Journal of Continuing Education in Nursing 28(3): 102–114

Davidson D 1998 Quality: an everyday event. British Journal of Theatre Nursing 7(10): 28–32

Downs S 1995 Learning at work. Kogan Page, London

Erickson G 1996 Operating safely. British Journal of Theatre Nursing 6(5): 48

Ferguson J 1995 Development of a post operative pain service (1). British Journal of Theatre Nursing 5(7): 29–32

Glen S 1995 Towards a new model of nursing education. Nurse Education Today 15: 90–95

Handy C 1993 Understanding organisations, 4th edn. Penguin Books, London

Harris J 1996 Animating learning in teams. In: Boud D, Miller N (eds) Working with experience: animating learning. Routledge, London

Hart G, Rotem A 1995 The clinical learning environment: nurses' perceptions of professional development in clinical settings. Nurse Education Today 15: 3–10

Hood P 1995 Opportunities for a specialist practitioner and advanced nursing practice. British Journal of Theatre Nursing 5(11): 26–27

James C R, Clarke B A 1994 Reflective practice in nursing: issues and implications for nurse education. Nurse Education Today 14: 82–90

Kolb D 1984 Experiential learning experience as the source of learning and development. Prentice Hall, New Jersey

Le Var R M H 1996 NVQs in nursing, midwifery and health visiting: a question of assessment and learning? Nurse Education Today 16(2): 85–93

MacRae W 1996 The team approach to anaesthesia. British Journal of Theatre Nursing 6(4): 9–10

Mallik M 1998 The role of nurse educators in the development of reflective practitioners: a selective case study of the Australian and UK experience. Nurse Education Today 18: 52–63

Milligan F 1998 Defining and assessing competence: the distraction of outcomes and the importance of the educational process. Nurse Education Today 18: 273–280

Patterson D H 1973 Humanistic education. Prentice Hall, London

Preston R 1996 Anaesthesia – room for expanding nursing practice. British Journal of Theatre Nursing 6(6): 5–8

Quinn F M 1988 The principles and practice of nurse education, 2nd edn. Croom Helm, London

Rushin J, Thakrar R, Taylor E et al 1998 Teamwork in the operating department. British Journal of Theatre Nursing 7(11): 13–17

Studdy S, Nicol M, Fox-Hiley A 1994 Teaching and learning clinical skills. Part 2 Development of a teaching model and schedule of skills development. Nurse Education Today 14: 186–193

Varona L 1997 The perioperative nurse – carer or technician? British Journal of Theatre Nursing 7(8): 10–13

Webster C 1996 Managing in difficult situations. British Journal of Theatre Nursing 5(11): 11–15

Wicker P 1996 The extended roles of nurses in surgery – what are the boundaries? A report on sessions from the Association of Surgeons of Great Britain and Northern Ireland Annual Meeting, Glasgow, 22–24 May. British Journal of Theatre Nursing 6(5): 32–33

Wicker P 1997 Sacred cows and sound practice. British Journal of Theatre Nursing 7(7): 31–34

Williams M 1995 Managing quality. British Journal of Theatre Nursing 5(2): 18–19

Williams M 1996 Managing continuing education. A consumer's and provider's point of view. Quay Books, Salisbury

Williams M 1997 Growing quality trees. Paper presented to the World Conference of Operating Room Nurses, 8–12 September, Toronto, Canada

Index

Page numbers in **bold** type refer to illustrations and tables